# BREAKFAST, LUNCH, and DINNER of CHAMPIONS

# BREAKFAST, LUNCH, and DINNER of CHAMPIONS

## Star Athletes' Diet Programs for Maximum Energy and Performance

## Jane Wilkens Michael

QUILL

New York    1984

*To* R.E.M.

2232264

# Acknowledgments

My thanks and appreciation, first of all, to Alex Ward, Editor of the Living Section of *The New York Times,* whose idea this was to begin with. Then, of course, I wish to thank all the athletes, coaches, trainers, and specialists who were so helpful in this project through the giving of their time, thoughts, and energy. Special thanks go to Steve Parker, Ken Schields, Bob Williams, Dr. James Whittam of the Shaklee Corporation, Don Gambril, Al Domenico, Roosevelt Sanders, Jr., Ronnie Barnes, Bill Fink, Jim Warfield, Gene Monahan, Bob Breunig, Dr. Robert Haas, Dr. Casey Clarke, and the staff at the Olympic Training Center in Colorado Springs. Also, Larry Fleischer of the NBA Players Assn., Ed Croke of the New York Giants, Peggy Gossit of the WTA, Les Wagner of the Islanders, Ed Stanton, Minute Maid, M&M Mars, ProServ's Jerry Solomon, the Nick Bollettieri Tennis Academy, David Ogrean and Paul Slagle of ESPN, June Silver, Steve Wainwright, and Michael Barnet. Not to mention my sons Alex and Philip for being so good while I was working. Finally, my gratitude to Alison Brown Cerier for making this all possible.

# Contents

# CHAPTER ONE

# Sports and Nutrition

In hockey, it's: "If it moves, hit it. If it doesn't, hit someone into it." Football coaches are given to saying: "If you can kneel you can crawl, if you can crawl you can stand, if you can stand you can walk, and if you can walk you can run. So get up, sucker, and run!" Or, the more straightforward, "When the going gets tough, the tough get going." Every sport has its equivalent proverb that all it takes is "guts," "intestinal fortitude," "the winning attitude," and "giving 110 percent" to be a success. But remember Julie Moss, who after bicycling 112 miles, swimming nearly two and a half miles, and running over twenty-six miles, had a big lead in the Ironman Triathlon Championship (women's division) only to collapse fifty yards from the finish line? She still managed to crawl across the line—for second place. Moss certainly was not short on guts. What she did lack, however, were those last few calories of blood sugar.

No coach has ever fined a player for arriving at training camp with too much attitude. On the other hand, Lou Piniella was docked a thousand dollars a day until he lost the eight pounds he had put on over the winter. Yankee owner George Steinbrenner felt (and Piniella ultimately agreed) that his player could perform better if he was thinner. A more dramatic case involved Dave Young, touted as the New York Giants' tight end of the future. He became a player of the past because he never met the weight limits set for him by the coaching staff. Today, an athlete's personal diet is as important as his or her agent. If the image of a successful professional athlete restricting his diet to half a cow and a keg of beer was ever true, it certainly is not any longer.

Denis Potvin, the dominating defenseman and captain of the Islanders, the only American hockey team to win the Stanley Cup four years in a row, is typical of the top modern competitor who has very defined ideas about nutrition. Potvin usually avoids red meat and finds that chicken, fish, fresh fruits and vegetables, and potatoes or spaghetti are all he needs. However, when he wants to increase his brute strength, he'll eat a rare steak. Mark Gastineau, an All-Pro member of the Jets' Sack Exchange, is another physical player who is extremely careful at the dinner table. Two of his rules are sticking to a high protein diet and staying away from sugar and starch. He won't even eat bread. Across the line from Mark, the New York Giants' huge (six feet six inch, 275 lb.) right tackle Gordon King is big on fruits and gets most of his protein from fish, eggs, and tofu. A red meat eater is Marvelous Marvin Hagler, who will have a steak and spaghetti between weigh-in and bout. On the other hand, the equally fearsome battler, linebacker Lawrence Taylor, has only a glass of orange juice on the day of a game. The diets of these and other sports superstars vary dramatically, from slender tennis powerhouse Ivan Lendl, who is a big meat eater, to one of basketball's premier power forwards, Maurice Lucas, who eats almost no meat. And whether it's New York Yankee Dave Winfield's sunflower seeds or Boston Celtic Scott Wedman's bee pollen (not to mention Ft. Lauderdale Striker Thomas Rongen's Siberian ginseng), they all have their secrets and theories. So do their coaches and trainers, from the Philadelphia 76ers' Al Domenico to boxing legend Angelo Dundee, to Mike Gallagher, coach of the U.S. Men's Cross-Country Ski Team.

These superstars are just some of those who have found

something important in their diets to maintain the highest levels in their performance. But performance is not the same for every athlete. For a free-style swimmer, it simply means swimming faster, but for a decathlete, it is obviously much more complex.

## The Role of Nutrition in Sports

A boxer's opponent is selected according to his weight. Too much weight and he may lose his title. Of course, if adding the weight is right for him, he will continue his success. Wilfred Benitez, for example, kept growing and won, successively, the junior welterweight (up to 140 lbs.), welterweight (up to 147 lbs.), and junior middleweight (up to 154 lbs.) crowns before being emphatically stopped in his quest for the middleweight title. And if a certain Olympic light heavyweight (up to 175 lbs.) champ named Cassius Clay hadn't grown into 210-pound heavyweight Muhammad Ali, boxing history would have been *very* different. More weight isn't always better, though. If a pro halfback has too little, he may lose more than a job; he can lose his ribs. The bottom line is that an athlete's weight will affect the pull of gravity on him and how much resistance to an opposing force can be provided. Newton, not Knute Rockne, gave us these lessons. What and how much he eats, however, will determine his avoirdupois.

Stamina, speed, and power can all be traced directly to nutrition. Like any other engine, the body uses up energy in creating energy. While the human system is an efficient user of its raw materials, the feeling of fatigue during digestion is clear evidence of the effort the body expends in converting fuel into a form that can generate power. Of the natural functions that the human being performs voluntarily, sex may be more fun but digestion requires more calories each day. Precisely how much energy is used and how long the process takes is an important element in any sports activity.

The demands on the system of the sixty-yard dash are obviously different from those of the marathon. Nevertheless, virtu-

13

ally all athletes and experts do not have a large meal within a few hours of a game. The old idea of having a raw steak right before a match is now totally discredited. Even years ago, top athletes did know better. All-time hockey great Gordie Howe, for example, discovered the benefits of afternoon pancakes thirty years ago. He also advocates ground beef instead of steak on game days to ease digestion. His spiritual, if not physical, successor, Wayne "The Great" Gretzky, may be the lone holdout. He eats his way right into the game. But just as in each individual athlete's case, Wayne's diet is tailor-made to his needs.

Beyond the needs of the actual performance are the less obvious requirements of an athlete's nutrition. These include the right diet to prepare for a season and the necessary changes for off-season, training, and actual competition. The right vitamins, minerals, and combinations can also extend competitive life. Are there recommended foods to take or shun in traveling and through time changes? Which combinations of foods help the body assimilate nutrients into the bloodstream and which make its task more difficult? What are the best nutrients to keep the eyes sharp, the reflexes quick, and the knees flexible? (Brilliant third baseman Graig Nettles, for example, keeps eyes and reflexes sharp with ten thousand units a day of vitamin A.)

Obviously, the ability to "stab a hot liner" is less important to a writer than a Major Leaguer, but we all want to feel better and younger, and that's what attention to diet can do. But just as a finely tuned engine requires high octane to operate at peak performance, the athlete needs the best return for his dietary investment.

No single diet is perfect for every athlete. Each sport has different demands and within each sport different positions or specialties often require differing regimes. This book is devoted to the study of the most popular sports in America and how the athletes, coaches, trainers, and medical specialists feel about the right nutrition for them. Included are also diets prepared by coaches, trainers, and nutritionists. Anyone can adapt them to a particular situation, but they are especially targeted for high school and college coaches (and parents of young participants in sports) who want to know what the experts advise for their sports. What do the New York Giants serve at training camp? What do the Yankees recommend off-season? What did the skiers eat at the Olympic Village at Sarajevo? These diets and many more are set out meal by meal and day by day. But first, a brief overview of the particular demands of each sport:

## BASEBALL

Baseball players used to be fairly simple to analyze. There were big guys who caught, played first base, left or right field, and threw thunderous fast balls from the mound when they weren't at bat hitting home runs and very long singles. The smaller fellows played the infield and center field, hit short singles, doubles, and triples, and usually were adept at executing the hit and run, sacrifice bunt, and steal. From the mound, they would throw a curve, a screw ball, the occasiónal knuckle ball, or a moist variant that could have done one or all of the above.

Today the game is much more complex. Consider the pitcher. With the advent of the slider, forkball, split-finger fastball, knuckle curve, et al., junk ballers are throwing harder and power pitchers are throwing softer. Perhaps the biggest change came with the introduction of the relief pitcher. The iron man of yore is only found in teams that do not have a decent relief pitcher. No Major League team would be without one. Whether the reliever is a BB thrower like enormous Goose Gossage of San Diego or a finesse pitcher of Rollie Fingers's class, his job is to get anywhere from one out to two innings of work done. In addition, the reliever will never know if he has to pitch at all in any given game. Unlike the starter, who follows a fixed rotation of pitching every four or five days, a reliever may pitch two or three days in a row and then not again for a week or more.

The reliever's counterpart at bat is the American League's invention, the designated hitter. While keeping the pitchers from running the base paths on those rare occasions when they would have had a hit or walk, the designated hitter himself is the ultimate specialist. His total game activity may be reduced to a few futile swings of the bat and trots to and from the dugout. Not a fielder, he sits and waits his turn, and then only if his batsmanship is successful does he get a chance to try his luck on the bases. On the other hand, to watch Piniella come up cold and stroke a RBI double is to see an artist at work.

Add night games, artificial turf and a 162-game season, and the strains on a modern Major Leaguer are more intense than on those in Babe Ruth's day. What all baseball players share is a need to follow the pulse of the game. Baseball has far and away the highest ratio of periods of nonactivity to activity, even for the pitchers and catchers. Yet few activities in sports place as many physical demands as those on a starting power pitcher's body. A ninety-mile per hour fastball will cover the sixty feet six inches from the pitcher to the catcher in less than half a second. The strain on the shoulder and arm caused by a sore toe forcing a hitch in the motion can ruin a great career. And few sports make as few demands as those on a pinch hitter or designated hitter.

Steve Garvey, Dave Winfield, Pete Rose, Rod Carew, Nolan Ryan, Tom Seaver, and George Brett are a few of the greats who will tell us how they cope with differing stresses of their game, while Yankee trainer Gene Monahan and his Cleveland Indian counterpart Jim Warfield will provide general ideas and specific diets.

## FOOTBALL

No sport has as many rigidly defined positions as does football. From the almost genteel dropback quarterback to the violent world of an interior lineman, the positions in football require skills that vary immensely. In the upper echelons of football, certainly at the professional level and probably at the college level as well, the two-way player is a thing of the past. But you don't have to tell a defensive lineman or cornerback on a team that has little offense that football can be a game of stamina. It is also a game where excellence is rewarded by extra attention. A slugger in baseball may get pitched around and a hot man in basketball may be fronted to keep the ball away from him, but top football players have the pleasure of double teaming. It may be an honor to have to fight off blocks of two 250-pound offensive linemen instead of just one, but it's an accolade many defensive stars would be willing to live without.

The positions on a football team break down into four main categories. First, there are the speed positions. Wide receivers, cornerbacks and safeties, and most halfbacks are successful with a combination of pure speed, body control and hand-to-eye coordination. The linebackers and fullbacks make up an intermediate class of athletes who need good speed yet sufficient power and upper body strength to be transitional players. They have to be able to move quickly in the open field and also be effective physically in short yardage situations. The interior linemen on the offense and defense require quickness (but not speed) and significant strength throughout their frames. To be able to withstand punishing contact for an entire game also means body weight distributions very different from that of the speed back. Finally, the professional or college quarterback in a pro-type offense usually does not require speed but needs quick feet to set up to pass, great hand-to-eye coordination, and a flexible body able to withstand hard tackles while in a relatively defenseless posture. Punters and placekickers require similar attributes, with the emphasis on strong legs and foot-to-eye coordination.

The other aspect of football that needs to be considered is the enormous range of weather conditions. No other sport attempts to pursue the same type and level of play in conditions ranging from Miami Septembers to Green Bay Decembers. Do the teams alter their diets depending on the season and locale? Should they?

Football's association with diet is longstanding; after all, it is the sport that gave us the "training table." It is what the players eat from and away from this supply source that is interesting. Lawrence Taylor, "Mean" Joe Greene, Anthony Munoz, Ed "Too Tall" Jones, Terry Bradshaw, Danny White, Tommy Kramer, Herschel Walker, Walter Payton, Dwight Clark, Redskin trainer Bubba Tyre, and others will discuss their diets and nutritional philosophies. Cowboys' conditioning coach Bob

17

Ward will add theory, and the New York Giants will provide their training camp menu.


## BASKETBALL

Basketball may well be the other extreme from baseball in regard to the amount of exertion required over time as compared to the amount of inactivity. In a well-played game with few fouls, the five players on each side are in motion almost constantly for the twelve-minute professional quarters or the twenty-minute college halves. Whether the team believes in the fast break or run-and-gun offense, or in a patterned set play approach, a good basketball player should always be on the move. Moving without the ball distinguishes the good team player from the individualist. Setting picks and screens and getting in position to receive a pass is the mental part of basketball. Being able to generate the energy for these activities in addition to running up and down the court on each change of possession is the physical part. A great basketball player combines the body control of a gymnast or ballet dancer with the speed of a sprinter, the jumping ability of a high jumper, the physical strength for rebounding of a linebacker, and the hand-to-eye coordination of a marksman. That may be why in recent years that ballplayer also has the bank account of a Texas oilman.

Basketball, too, has seen a modern era of specialization. No longer are there just two big forwards, a huge center, and a pair of relatively petite guards. The game now witnesses power forwards, small forwards, point or playmaking guards, and off or shooting guards. And today's guards are often taller than were the forwards on championship teams of yesterday. Nevertheless, the dynamics of basketball require similar physical acts irrespective of position. Guards, centers, and forwards all have to play offense and defense alternately. They have to be able to run, jump, and bump into other players. The differences in ball handling and shooting, as well as how high they jump and how fast they run, relate more to individual talent than positional

18

requirements. The small forward and off guard are hard to distinguish in a fluid offense and the power forward and center play similar roles. The question for all basketball players is how to keep up their energy levels through a grueling season while getting the most out of their talent. The search for an answer has caused many players to seek unusual diets. For example, Walt "Clyde" Frazier in his All-Pro days with the Knicks ate steamed spinach with brown rice and sesame seeds, washed down by a glass of spinach, carrot, and celery juice before each game. And John "Hondo" Havlicek's secret was to come into training camp ten pounds underweight. These two superstars plus the diets of Adrian Dantley, Willis Reed, Marvin Webster, Kareem Abdul-Jabbar, and more, are the heart of the basketball chapter, while Al Domenico, trainer of the Philadelphia 76ers, will tell you how to have the energy of a pro.

## ICE HOCKEY

Ice hockey legends concerning the toughness of its athletes abound. Toothless grins are almost a badge of honor. Hockey creates the greatest potential violence in sports. In no other situation do you have 200 pound opponents carrying deadly sticks and hurtling at each other at great speed with the intent to make contact. This is above and beyond the fisticuffs, elbowing, and tripping that are an intrinsic part, unfortunately, of the sport.

Hockey does have three distinct groups of players—forwards, defensemen, and goalies. In general, goalies live by their reflexes, defensemen by their physiques, and forwards by their speed and agility. All require phenomenal hand-to-eye coordination to deal with the puck.

The goalie's job description is simple. He stands in a closely prescribed area waiting for a hard black object to be hurtled at him from any distance at speeds up to a hundred miles an hour. He is far and away the most heavily armored sportsman. The defensemen are his main line of support. They must use their bodies and sticks to block the opposing forwards and/or the incoming puck. The great ones also have the offensive talents of a forward, being able to maneuver at great speed and fire a bullet to the opposing goal, but the offense is supposed to be in the hands of the forwards, center, and wings. Their job is to bring the attack, albeit weaving and passing and shooting at great speed, and it's all done on a bed of ice.

While we noted that basketball required the most continuous activity by its individual participants, hockey is significantly faster moving because of the pace at which the skaters and the puck can cover the larger distances of the hockey rink. The speed is maintained by constant substitutions, usually every one to two minutes of actual playing time.

Accordingly, a hockey player needs to be able to put out total effort for one to two minutes and then rest for longer periods while his teammates carry the load. Detroit Red Wings veteran defenseman Brad Park copes by drinking three or four cups of black coffee (a natural stimulant) and eating a chocolate bar an hour and a half before each game. Three or four beers replace fluids and vitamin $B_6$ afterwards. The Islanders' perennial All-Star center Bryan Trottier, on the other hand, staunchly avoids chocolate and all alcoholic beverages. Yet, the other aspects of their diets are surprisingly similar. The same cannot be said for Gordie Howe and Mike Bossy, or Wayne Gretzky and anyone. Their diets and those of Bobby Clarke, Chico Resch, Barry Beck, and others will reveal the cold weather, high energy life of hockey players, while Rangers trainer Bob Williams will add his thoughts on nutrition and a model regime.


SOCCER

The world's most popular team sport is what we call soccer and everyone else calls football. It, too, has evolved towards specialization, away from the traditional goalie, defenseman, midfielder, and forward to such strange beasts as sweepers, strikers, and *liberos*. The result has been more fluid offenses and more complex defenses. From a differentiation between defensive and offensive players proved similiar to that found in hockey, it is now more like basketball's difference between forwards and guards, i.e., the talents are approximately the same, the variations being in the roles played rather than the skill required. Of course, given the size of the arena and the ten players per side that may be involved in an attack, there is greater role separation in soccer than in basketball. For example, other than in a penalty or corner kick situation, a fullback finds it much more difficult to get in a scoring position than would any basketball player.

Extraordinary stamina and thunderous leg strength are the requirements for excellence in all ten field positions. The goalie, of course, needs very different skills. Besides being the only player needing hand-to-eye instead of foot-to-eye coordination, he also requires great reflexes and body control.

The rules of the game would seem to indicate greater individual effort to stay in motion then does basketball. However, since the ball is much more difficult to move accurately by foot than hand, and given the longer distances involved, plays in soccer tend to develop more slowly. Therefore, moving without the ball on offense to create scoring opportunities has to be more patient and controlled. In addition, the lengthier playing times and limited substitutions require the player to pace himself. The great players have the ability to combine stamina and bursts of sudden energy. To see a Giorgio Chinaglia or Paolo Rossi spend sixty or seventy minutes maneuvering constantly in spontaneous or preset patterns, even though not at full speed, can be mesmerizing. It is exactly at that moment when the defender is being worn into weakness or lack of concentration that a quick pass turns the mongoose into a cobra striking a bullet from foot or head at the helpless goalie.

Aside from the physical aspects of the game itself, soccer, being such an international sport, also requires the ability to play despite traveling great distances throughout the world. And unlike tennis, for example, the players usually do not have enough time to adjust to the changes in hour or diet before the critical performances are required. Anyone who has had to make a business trip can appreciate the problem of needing all of your faculties after a major dislocation. One man who has traveled the world over playing an unequalled level of midfield play is Franz Beckenbauer. He copes by skipping breakfast and having a larger lunch instead on the day of travel. Besides Beckenbauer, Chinaglia, and Rossi, we'll hear from American stars Ricky Davis, Glen Myernick and Dan Canter plus NASL international greats like Brian Kidd and Wim Rijsbergen. Ft. Lauderdale Strikers trainer Ray Jaffet will provide insights, and Ken Schields, Tampa Bay's trainer, will add an entire primer on soccer nutrition.


## TENNIS

Certainly no group of athletes covers a circuit more far-flung than that of the top flight tennis player. Australian and Western European tournaments are as important as any in the United States. And while they don't have to face the climate of an outdoor December football game, certainly the dietary concerns and ability to maintain conditioning must vary between playing in Madison Square Garden in the winter and on the hot clay of Roland Garros in the summer.

While individual athletes, whether male or female, may have different strengths in their game, the basic attributes of hand-to-eye coordination, quick reflexes, a strong arm, and fast feet are needed by all tennis players. The mixture of skills for a particular athlete will determine the style of play—serve and volley versus baseline, for example—but real success requires them all. It is also a sport that demands longevity in an unparalleled manner considering the exertion required. While Mean Joe Greene is now knocking out commercials instead of opposing halfbacks, much older Pancho Segura is still spending hours on the court playing and teaching.

The key is to maintain the fitness of tournament players throughout their schedule, and to allow weekend warriors to maximize their performance. To that end, Chris Evert Lloyd has found that for her pasta plays an important role in supplying complex carbohydrates. And Martina Navratilova credits a special low protein and fat diet in helping her overcome a long slump. Their diets plus those of Billie Jean King, Ivan Lendl, Gene Mayer and others will serve as a prologue to former WCT trainer Steve Parker's instructive—and hilarious—memoirs.

## SWIMMING

Another sport whose habitués have had to adjust to moving indoors over the winter is swimming. Swimming may be the most purely physical activity, using virtually every muscle group at all times. It is also a very basic sport. Other than the initial dive or start and the turns at the end of the pool, it is simply an exercise of executing the relevant stroke more perfectly and faster than the competition. Top conditioning is absolutely essential. The swimmer's understanding of how his or her body works, of how to generate the maximum output of energy while avoiding such obvious dangers as stomach cramps, may be more important than for any other athlete. But of course, differences will exist because of the various distances that competitive swimmers strive for. The short sprints require a burst of energy, while the longer races require sustained production. Perhaps most interesting are the middle distances, which take much longer in swimming than in running. Do the top athletes prepare for the two hundred meter breaststroke in the same way that a runner trains for the two hundred yard dash or the mile run? Montreal Olympic stars John Naber and Wendy Boglioli, along with the 1984 crop of top Olympic swimmers, their coaches, and Don Gambril, the coach of the Olympic Men's Swimming Team, will divulge some of their secrets.

## SKIING

Skiing provides dramatic variations in speed. In the same way that the sixty yard dash and the marathon may well be different sports, downhill skiing and cross-country skiing have little in common besides snow and the idea of traversing it on two runners. Alpine skiing, whether slalom, grand slalom, or straight

23

downhill, is the sport for lovers of speed. Only sky diving projects the human body through greater accelerations and sustained velocity without the use of mechanical assistance. Body control at high speed is what counts, a combination of flexibility and power. This, of course, must be dealt with in the high altitudes and frigid weathers of the snow-bound sport. Triple Olympic champion Jean-Claude Killy, for one, found that high protein foods like chicken and fish are important to fight the cold.

The demands of Nordic skiing are quite different. Much closer to long distance running and swimming, cross-country requires fluidity in motion and stamina. Upper body strength is considerably more important as a propellant than in downhill skiing. And strength, pure and simple, in the legs becomes more crucial to performance than that in the muscle groups necessary to guide the downhill skier in holding to an aerodynamic position. Anyone who has had to shovel a walk in winter will appreciate the skills of Bill Koch, America's Cross-Country Skiing World Cup Champion, who can cover thirty miles while you're doing the driveway.

Killy's and Koch's diet tips, plus those of Cindy Nelson and the U.S. Men's and Women's Olympic coaches, will provide practical advice, while the Shaklee Corporation, the official nutrition consultant to the U.S. Ski Team, will add some heavyweight scientific support, the Winter Olympics' diet and some pointed tips for weekend skiers.


BOXING

Not all boxers can float like a butterfly and sting like a 105-millimeter howitzer, but they all wish they could. And while clearly the art of avoiding being concussed is an important attribute, the concept of the untrained, unskilled dockworker able to succeed as a boxer is totally outdated, if indeed it was ever valid. Superb hand-to-eye coordination and hand speed, power throughout the body and agility mark the great boxer. One need only remember the Thrilla' in Manila to exemplify the kind of stamina that a great boxer must have.

On top of this, unlike nearly all other athletes, the boxer (and wrestler) must know his weight to the pound. Fluctuation from one pound to the next may result in fighting someone five pounds lighter instead of forty pounds heavier, if there is a slip into the heavyweight class. Even at lower classes, the difference between the lightest of the lower weights and the heaviest of the next higher weight can be drastic in trying to out-muscle an opponent over even the three rounds of international amateur boxing. As in other contact sports, the good small man may be able to fend off the less talented larger man, but he is going to be woefully outmatched against the good big man. Remember, modern boxing gloves protect the wearer's hands much more than the opponent's features. Muhammad Ali used his amazing agility to keep his face unmarred, but maintained his endurance while controlling his weight through a special diet devised by comedian and health food fanatic Dick Gregory. His great opponent, Smokin' Joe Frazier, now passes on his nutritional know-how to his sons and nephews. Their diets as well as that of more recent great world champions Larry Holmes, Marvelous Marvin Hagler, Wilfred Benitez and Donald Curry share center ring with the advice of all-time great trainers Angelo Dundee and Cus D'Amato and their current competitors.

## RUNNING

Jogging has caught the American public's fancy unlike any other sport. Even so, it is basically the duffer's equivalent of long distance running. But the marathon, the pinnacle of these endeavors, showed at its conception just how much stress it can cause on the human body in the run that gave it its name nearly twenty-five hundred years ago. Upon completing his message that Athens was saved from the Persians, after having run twenty-six and a quarter miles from Marathon, Pheidippides died of exhaustion. Nowadays, a severe case of blisters is the most common ailment, but for the tough competitor and the overzealous novice as well, drastic dehydration is still the recompense for unrealistic goals.

Running as a sport, however, is much more than the marathon. At the other extreme are the short dashes, sixty yards indoors, one hundred yards outdoors. The muscular and general physiological demands are totally different for those regimes even though they still entail just moving the body by foot over a track through a distance. As in swimming, the specialties break down into three areas: sprints, middle distance, and long distance. Once again, the concepts of quick energy versus slow burning stamina or trying to achieve a workable compromise between the two become all-important. Mary Decker, the world's premier middle distance runner and the 1982 Sullivan Award laureate as the best amateur athlete in the United States, for instance, alters her normally balanced diet to load up on bread, potatoes, and hot cereal four hours before she races. We'll also hear from Bill Rogers, Rod Dixon, and other stars on their regimes, plus some in-depth advice from the Human Performance Lab at Ball State University, and a vegetarian weight *gain* diet from Dick Gregory.

Stamina, speed, power, coordination, agility, consistency, and stress are all parts of the sports world. An athlete's ability to master some or all of these will determine his or her success. The body can only get away with certain splurges and excesses for a while. Even a teenager should maximize the life of talent by starting early with the right training and nutrition. Certainly mature athletes have to know better—and the successful ones do.

CHAPTER TWO

# Nutrition and Sports

Why ask athletes about nutrition? For those of us who barely have enough stamina to cross a crowded room, climb a long flight of stairs, or mow the lawn, who better to ask for their energy secrets? Athletes who have to ski miles cross-country, run up and down a basketball court or a soccer field, not to mention go fifteen rounds with Muhammad Ali are people who need maximum energy, even to keep going when they don't feel like it.

Everyone has mornings when they feel so tired that they just don't want to go to work, but in most cases the work involves going to an office and sitting. Imagine if you had to play four hours of grueling championship tennis feeling this way. What would you do? And even office work involves days when you need that little bit extra. If there is a big meeting with the boss, is it better to have eaten a large bowl of spaghetti the night before or to have an extra cup of coffee that morning? Should breakfast be large or light?

Top athletes are tested daily. They need to know what works for them and what doesn't. And the people who train and coach them have to keep current on all the ideas about performance-related nutrition. The tips and secrets they divulge represent the latest concepts in healthful eating. And athlete fuel is our fuel too, so their ideas can help us. Weekend sportsmen and women as well as novice athletes can learn from the pros how to avoid heat exhaustion and cramps, what to eat to gain, lose, or maintain weight, both when you are physically active and when you are not, or what foods will provide peak energy when you need it. The livelihoods of the superstars of sports are dependent upon their knowing the answers, and answers are what this book is all about.

First, however, to better understand both the questions and the answers, it is necessary to know the language of nutrition, from alpha tocopherol to zinc. In the ensuing chapters we will hear sundry advice from various athletes and halth practitioners that will at times be couched in technical phrases. Rather than constantly repeat a lengthy explanation of the concepts, here is a brief review of the whys and wherefores.

## Ground Rules

The first thing to remember is that while athletic champions may be demigods to their fans, they are still *Homo sapiens.* There are certainly very good reasons aside from any dietary differences as to why I cannot run as fast as Mary Decker or why my husband would not survive very long trying to block Lawrence Taylor. Under all that exceptional ability, however, athletes are people too. The point is that good nutrition for a competitive athlete has the same roots as for a housewife, lawyer, author, plumber, secretary, or accountant. Making appropriate allowances for the intensity of activity, and age or sex differences, the best advice for athletes tends to be the best advice for all the rest of us.

The most abused aspect of nutritional guidance, though, is the tendency to take results of observations and experiments that determine a norm and apply them willy-nilly to any individual. No diet, no matter how famous the author or how elegant the neighborhood it purports to represent, will work for everyone. For example, a calorie is the amount of energy needed to raise the temperature of one kilogram (2.2 pounds) of pure water by one degree centigrade (1.8° Fahrenheit). A gram of protein and a gram of carbohydrates each provides four calories, while a gram of fat produces nine. But if one or another of a vast variety of circumstances occurs, the ability of an individual to utilize that energy can be impaired. To put it another way, as far as calories are concerned, it is not what you put in your mouth but what your body uses that counts.

Only in a perfect world with perfect people would everyone be able to eat exactly the same things and get the same benefits. The orthodox dietary guidance that complete meals including all the basic foods are all anyone needs to be in peak condition ignores individual variations. Some of the more straightforward reasons why a single diet will not suit everyone are the following:

• Genetically derived dispositions can alter body chemistries in a myriad of ways from metabolic rate to ability to digest certain foods. A common example of this is a shortage of the enzyme lactase which is needed to break down lactose, the sugar found in milk. While not very common in infants, it becomes almost normal for adults to have some degree of lactase shortage. We all know someone who cannot tolerate dairy products, and this is why.
• Physical trauma and physiological disabilities can result from injuries, diseases, overindulgence, pollution, or even malnutrition. Probably the greatest source of physical difficulty in American adults is poor nutrition. Obesity and hypertension go hand in hand as both symptoms and results.
• Finally, and perhaps that which has an overriding effect on many, is psychological stress. Besides the extreme problem of mental imbalances and some resulting physical manifestations such as anorexia nervosa, moderate stress has a direct physical effect on digestion, the cardiovascular system, and many other body functions.

Next, there are the differences relating to actual calorie usage. Marathon swimmers, runners and skiers, basketball and soccer players, and boxers are examples of athletes with enormous energy needs in training and competition. Downhill skiers and sprinters, football, baseball, and hockey players are all characterized by the intensity of their exertion. The body can use only a certain amount of calories at a time, no matter how hard one works, so these sports need fewer gross calories but more "peak" calories. When applying an athlete's advice to others, these special needs have to be considered. Similarly, people with higher metabolic rates burn up calories faster because their bodies' chemical reactions convert fuel to energy more quickly. One lesson is to choose your sport by whether your metabolic rate allows you to store and use the energy required for endurance sports.

Basic nutritional concepts applied to one's general health and circumstances do provide valuable assistance in evaluating your dietary lifestyle. The only caveat is to keep in mind the differences. The best way to make certain that you're on the right track (literally and figuratively) with a significant change in diet is to have a nutritionist advise you, preferably after observation and testing, including a complete blood analysis.

# Food for Action

Carbohydrates, fats, and protein are the energy sources in the human diet. Everything else that we eat only assists the body in processing and using these three. The first two provide fuel in the ordinary course, while protein is both the clay from which the bricks are made and an emergency fuel reserve.

## CARBOHYDRATES

Of the three, this is the only one with an accurately descriptive name. "Carbohydrate" is simply the chemical name for molecules composed of carbon, hydrogen and oxygen. When nutritionists speak of carbohydrates, though, they are referring to only three basic forms that appear naturally in our diet—sugars, starches, and fibers.

Pure sugar is found in six varieties. Glucose, otherwise known as dextrose or blood sugar, is the form actually used in the bloodstream for nourishment. Sucrose is far and away the biggest source of sugar in the American diet. Derived from sugar cane and sugar beets, it appears traditionally as white, refined table sugar, and brown and confectioner's sugar. Fructose is, as its name suggests, the form of sugar found naturally in fruit. Surprisingly, it tends to taste considerably sweeter than sucrose. Lactose is milk sugar and is much less sweet than sucrose. It is converted into the fifth form of sugar, galactose, which is not otherwise commonly found in nature. Finally, there is maltose, the basic sugar in most cereals and grains.

Sugar provides quick energy because it is either already in the form to enter the bloodstream or can be readily converted into glucose without complicated chemical reactions. But plain sugar has no vitamins, no protein, no minerals, enzymes, or anything else. That is why it is often referred to as having empty calories. And if the energy is not immediately needed, since the sugar goes so quickly into the bloodstream, it cannot be used or retained in its present form and must be converted to fat for storage. Since the body can make glucose for energy from more complex carbohydrates as well as all fats and protein, nutritionists recommend eating foods that bring more to the body than just glucose.

Foods high in starches are the good guys among the carbohydrates, contrary to their traditional reputation. Whole grains and potatoes, almost pariahs in the diet menus of not too long ago, have made a striking comeback. Starches are merely a very complex form of carbohydrate, chemically similar to sugar. However, because of its structure a starch is much more difficult for the body to process. Therefore, it does not rush into the bloodstream and it burns much more slowly. One benefit is that blood sugar levels do not have to be stabilized by a sharp insulin injection from the pancreas, which either converts the excess into fat or forces it out of the system entirely. (It is this role of

31

insulin in controlling the level of glucose in the bloodstream that goes awry in diabetes. Sugar is normally bad for diabetics because it puts too much of a strain on the already imperfect system.) Fruits and vegetables share the same virtue to a lesser extent. They also require more digestion to produce their fructose, glucose, or maltose, but less than the starches. Only when the bareboned sugar is served is the process accelerated, causing what some nutritionists feel are artificial highs and rollercoaster blood chemistry.

The training technique of carbohydrate loading is based on the biological way that muscle tissue stores extra energy in the form of glycogen. Glycogen is a very close chemical cousin of glucose and can be converted to glucose in the muscles for extra energy merely by adding water molecules. Loading carbohydrates lengthens endurance by increasing muscular glycogen content, instead of increasing either fat elsewhere in the body, which can be drawn on more slowly, or blood sugar levels (or the quantity of fatty acids in the blood which combine with oxygen molecules to the same effect) which dissipate more quickly. To load carbs, starting about a week before the targeted event, a normal or even slightly low carbohydrate diet is maintained. About three days prior to the match, exercise is reduced and the consumption of carbohydrates is highly increased. The result is a greater amount of glycogen in the muscle tissue. Some tests have indicated that stamina can be increased by up to 300 percent in activities requiring sustained effort over periods in excess of thirty minutes to an hour or more. Generally, muscles that are not forced to strain over a lengthy period of time will run on the blood sugar and fatty acids that move through the tissue. Only when stress increases and the muscle cannot restore itself from its normally available supplies does it dip into the stored glycogen. This is consumed until the muscle is exhausted, which results from a total lack of fuel or a blocking accumulation of the waste products (primarily lactic acid) caused by the burning up of the glucose.

Whether it comes from sugars or starches, glucose is the primary fuel for muscular activity, which is of course paramount in all athletic endeavors. The body requires less energy and fewer additional nutrients to convert a carbohydrate into glucose than either protein or fats. And the best foods are those that nature provides with all the paraphernalia the body needs to process carbohydrate content into glucose. For example, whole grains (but not refined flour or polished rice) include significant doses of the B complex vitamins which are required to convert starches into energy-delivering form, as well as bran to help the body eliminate waste materials left after the glucose has been removed.

Bran is perhaps the best known form of fiber, the third type of carbohydrate, but it is certainly not the only one. Fibers share one property—the difficulty which the human gastrointestinal tract has in breaking them down. The hallmark of fiber is that virtually the only digestion is done by the bacteria in the large intestine. Unfortunately, another fact about fiber is that it is the substance that an incredible proportion of American foods have refined, processed or boiled out.

Fibers come in various chemical forms, the best known being cellulose, the stuff that makes things like apples and celery crisp. Usually, but not always, they are very hygroscopic, i.e., they absorb moisture without dissolving. Since fibers pass through the system without being broken down, they fill up the digestive tract ·without providing any usable calories, thereby giving the feeling of fullness while taking excess water out of the system and preventing cramping and colonic irritation by giving the intestines something to play with long after the meal. For these reasons, high fiber diets have recently been very much in vogue.

To the athlete, foods very high in fiber have two disadvantages. First of all, as noted, they are relatively low in usable calories and will not provide a quick burst of blood sugar or significant glucose or glycogen over a longer period. In addition, due to their susceptibility to attack by intestinal bacteria, fibrous foods are likely to provoke a gas attack while being digested. That is why so many athletes who use high fiber diets shift to nonfibrous carbohydrates, like pasta, shortly before a game or match. It is rather tough to punt when you are doubled over in pain.

## FATS

First the good news. Fats have more than twice (nine to four) the energy potential per gram than carbohydrates or protein. They are also composed of much more complex molecular structures* than carbohydrates (although they are also composed only of carbon, hydrogen, and oxygen) and are therefore digested more slowly, leaving a longer feeling of satisfaction and providing more sustained energy. Many athletes avoid all desserts and sweets but admit to a weakness for ice cream. That may be for a good reason they don't realize—that high fat ice cream forces the body to slow down its absorption of the sugar also found in it to give a double dose of slow burning energy. The second most common "sin" is chocolate, which also mixes fat, in the form of oils, with sugar.

Once stored in the body, fats act as insulation between the skin and the internal organs and play an important role in protecting the internal organs from damage in activities with a lot of physical contact. In other words, while a long distance runner might not need body fat, a cross-country skier should have some for insulation and a football or hockey player needs a good deal more. Dietary fats also help certain digestive and circulatory functions. One of their components, linoleic acid, is essential for the formation of body fat and is also believed to be important for beautiful skin and shiny hair. Furthermore, certain vitamins and other essential nutrients are not water soluble and are only dissolved in fats.

The bad news about fats is that most Americans are eating the wrong kinds of fats. At the heart of fat molecular structures are three types of molecules known as saturated, monounsaturated, and polyunsaturated fatty acids. The three groups are distinguished by the bonding between or among the carbon atoms. The distinction on the store or kitchen shelf is that fats made of saturated fatty acids are solid at room temperature while the others tend to be liquid. Olive oil, peanut oil, corn and

---

*Actually triglycerides, organic esters produced by the chemical substitution of three of the hydrogen atoms in glycerin by acid radicals, if you really want to know.

safflower oil are chemical cousins to lard, identical other than at the fatty acid stage. Unsaturated molecules can readily combine with other molecules, while saturated ones are complete and generally closed off. The hydrogenated fats used in products like margarine to convert liquids to solids is merely hydrogen added to an unsaturated fatty acid. The disadvantage of unsaturated fats is that additional oxygen can readily combine with the molecules to render them saturated, but in so doing they become rancid, no longer digestible. Once again, though, nature comes to its own aid. Most natural forms of polyunsaturated fats are also concentrated sources of vitamins C and E which are effective anti-oxidants; in other words, they prevent oxygen from bonding with molecules and turning them rancid.

From these basic scientific facts, we come to the dispute over cholesterol. Cholesterol, a member of the alcohol family, is essential to good cell health in all tissues because of its role in the building of cell membranes, in the formation of hormones and vitamin D and in the digestion of fats. It also is considered to be the prime mover in many forms of heart disease because it is often the main element in the deposits that block arteries, leading to reduced blood flow, hypertension, and various coronary diseases. Since the human liver produces quite a bit of cholesterol from other substances in food, we do not seem to need any additional cholesterol in our diet. Excess cholesterol has to be moved out of the bloodstream to avoid its eventually depositing on arterial walls. This is accomplished naturally by a form of protein known as lipoprotein (literally, a fat protein). There are good or high density lipoproteins and bad or low and very low density ones. The latter seem to keep the cholesterol from being eliminated from the system while the former help the body keep it under control. Tests indicate that polyunsaturated fats increase the amount of high density lipoproteins and decrease the others, while saturated fats have the opposite effect.

Milk, butter, cheese, egg yolks, and red meat are the main sources of saturated fats in the American diet. Just naming that list explains why we consume too much of them. On the other hand, the good fat component, linoleic acid, is found in the highest percentages in such American non-staples as safflower oil and sunflower oil. Also, while red meat and poultry tend to have saturated fats, fish does not.

Fat appears to be less a threat and more a boon for athletes than for their more sedentary friends. Since they have a greater caloric need, the extra energy resulting from the higher caloric content per gram is welcome. In addition, strenuous exercise helps keep the harmful cholesterol impact to a minimum by somehow increasing the level of friendly lipoproteins. On the other hand, anyone who is trying to lose body fat through exercising should know that each pound of body fat contains about thirty-five hundred calories of energy. That means that to lose one pound of that fat through diet or exercise one has to eat thirty-five hundred calories less than what is required to maintain your normal body weight and activity. To make matters worse, the body needs fewer calories to sustain fat (which basically just lies there) than muscle tissue. Just to break even, a person who has ten pounds of fat instead of muscle has to eat less than someone who has developed the muscle.


## PROTEINS

The sources of saturated fat in the American diet are far and away the most common forms of protein, mainly animal protein, but vegetables also contain considerable quantities. All living things are made up of those incredibly complicated strings of molecules, the basic ingredients of which are called amino acids. The main difference between the chemical make-up of protein and that of the carbohydrates and fats is that protein molecules are not limited to carbon, hydrogen, and oxygen. Protein also contains nitrogen (in fact, 'amino' is based on ammonia, a nitrogen-hydrogen compound) and some patterns have other components such as sulphur and phosphorus.

There are two kinds of amino acids, those the body produces itself and those that it can get only from food. The latter are called the essential amino acids. Most of the animal protein foods are complete protein sources, which means that they include all of the essential amino acids in addition to several others. A few of the vegetables which provide polyunsaturated fats are also complete, but usually vegetables must be combined with either animal protein or another vegetable to come up with all of them.

Since the chemical composition of proteins is different from carbohydrates and fats, the body cannot convert them into protein. On the other hand, excess protein can be stripped of its nitrogen and broken down into glucose when more ready sources are not available. Protein is not an efficient source of energy because of the effort the body must expend to extract its calories. It provides four calories per gram versus the nine in fats, and also causes greater strain than extracting the four calories per gram from carbohydrates. Also, the body needs to eliminate the leftover nitrogen. This is accomplished by creating urea and uric acid, in which form it is eliminated in the fashion their names suggest. While that's great if you're creating fertilizer, it isn't any use to the body and just requires the kidneys to work overtime. So ideally, you get your energy from carbohydrates and fats, and employ protein for what it is designed to do, which is virtually everything other than supplying energy. Protein is the building block for all the cells and tissues in the human system (and all other life forms), and is at the heart of almost all the other makers and shakers in the body. Enzymes are made from proteins, hormones are protein derivatives and our nails, hair, and nerve cells are all protein. Protein's forms and versatility far exceed the other basics, but the amount that a person needs each day is limited to the amount of those items that is broken down, injured, or needs to grow. The protein requirements of children and adolescents are therefore greater than those of adults. Flexing a muscle uses just glucose, not protein. However, putting muscle on, in training camp, general weight lifting or otherwise working out, requires a certain amount of additional protein. But except for the athlete who is putting on significant muscle tissue, the amount of extra protein needed is still probably far less than that in the average American's daily diet. The other type of athlete who may need extra protein is the one in a physical contact sport. If you are an interior lineman and every day, and certainly every game, you injure and slightly tear or break down muscle tissue, you need a steady diet of readily convertible protein to rebuild it.

In the American diet the real problem associated with protein is not that we eat too much protein, but that it carries excess baggage. The animal tissue that is the most common source of our protein, and especially red meats, is flavorful not because of protein, which by itself is dry and lifeless, but because of fat. The marbling in a fine steak is almost pure animal fat, nearly all saturated.

Extreme protein needs aside, the only other conceivable use of red meat by athletes is in sating the atavistic urge that is fulfilled by gorging on the flesh of our kill. The concept of the mean machine which thrives on raw steak is more psychological than physiological. For athletes who have to engage in gladiatorial combat, however, the haunting urges of a more physical past cannot be totally disregarded. But for others, in more finesse-related or cerebral pursuits, or for those who do not need subconscious urgings to hurl their bodies about, there are very few nutritional reasons for the amounts of red meat that appear in any American's diet, including an athlete's. Meat, poultry, eggs, and fish are probably needed only once a day, especially if they are eaten in association with vegetables that provide incomplete protein. Peas, beans (especially soy beans), peanuts, and seeds have the best vegetable protein along with whole grain wheat, rice, and corn. So a lot of spaghetti with a little meat sauce would be a good source of protein, as would a Chinese vegetarian dish that included peanuts and rice (although peanuts, like most other nuts, are quite high in fat, albeit mostly unsaturated fat). Clearly, the best sources of animal protein with the least amount of fat and cholesterol are turkey, chicken, and fish, and the white meat in the poultry is much better than the dark.

## Vitamins

The above discussion of the "big three" is noncontroversial even between orthodox nutritionists and health food fanatics. The same cannot be said for opinions on vitamins and minerals. The dispute ranges from the idea that a normal balanced diet should suffice without any supplements to the prescription of mega-doses. Vitamins (the name meaning life from ammonia, again going back to the nitrogen-hydrogen combinations that differentiate proteins from carbohydrates and fats) are indisputably essential for happy and healthy living. However, one expert's toxic overdose is another's essential supplement. People do not even agree on what substances constitute vitamins. There are certain standard ones, known usually by a letter of the alphabet, but there is substantial disagreement over others. Basically, a vitamin must be an organic substance that is necessary for proper functioning of one or the other of our systems. The key work is "necessary." If it is not necessary, the theory is that it should not be considered a vitamin whether or not it is merely useful, or just appears in the body with no as yet identified role. Since they are used in such minute quantities, and in the middle of such complicated chemical reactions inside the human body, until vivisection becomes a popular sport it remains very difficult to pinpoint exactly if and how vitamins and putative vitamins really work.

By and large, vitamins interact with enzymes. Enzymes are the catalysts of virtually every biochemical reaction from cellular to circulatory and digestive. True catalysts, they are not consumed in the reaction, but they do wear out and lose their potency after playing their role. Therefore, they need to be replaced from time to time. Some vitamins are produced in the body from other nutrients; others are taken in whole cloth from foods. In general, there is nothing the body needs in the way of vitamins (and minerals) that cannot be taken in the ordinary course in a balanced diet. Nevertheless, in recovering from an illness, in changing a diet (for instance in carbohydrate loading), and generally in reacting to any major physiological or psychological trauma, certain vitamins and minerals are needed in greater quantities. Unless the diet is very carefully planned to add rich sources of those vitamins and minerals, supplements are obviously the answer. The key is to carefully select from the myriad of choices the ones that suit the particular needs and not just grab one that has the most of everything. Freshness, sensibility in matching dosage to need, avoidance of sugar coatings, food coloring, and chemical additives, and perhaps, as discussed further on, chelation of minerals, should be checked.

## VITAMIN A

Eating carrots improves the eyesight because carotene is a base form of vitamin A from which the body produces the real thing. An alcohol, vitamin A is found in its final form in animals, especially in liver and eggs, and only in the carotene form in plants. As are all the vitamins except the B complex vitamins and vitamin C, it is not soluble in water, only in fat. Vitamin A is essential for seeing in dim and dark light, known as night vision, and has been associated with a wide variety of functions and deficiencies of the skin and all the linings of the digestive and respiratory systems. It is stored in the body, so temporary shortages in diet can be made up for, but it should be an important element in any dietary plan. Besides meat, dark green vegetables and deeply colored fruits are good sources. Grandma's favorite, cod liver oil, is also a very rich source of vitamin A.

Vitamin A is one of the most controversial megadose subjects. On one hand, megadoses have been claimed to cure a wide variety of diseases, and on the other, overdoses have been considered highly toxic.

## THE B COMPLEX VITAMINS

B complex is really a group of very different vitamins that have been popularly lumped together because they share their ability to be dissolved in water, are generally needed in converting food to energy, and tend to be found in the same foods. The individual B vitamins are the following:

*Thiamin, vitamin B₁* One of the typical casualties of refined flour, thiamin (meaning sulfur and ammonia) is found in wheat germ and whole grains, along with various peas and beans, liver and other organ meats, and brewer's yeast. Apparently it is a coenzyme, a material necessary to activate the work of an enzyme. In this case, $B_1$ helps the enzymes that break down carbohydrates into glucose. It is a classic case of nature providing its carbohydrates with the activator to help their digestion. Unfortunately, in refining and processing many of the carbohydrate sources, we eliminate the thiamin so the body has to look elsewhere. The classic $B_1$ deficiency is called beri beri; lesser shortages cause milder symptoms of that disease.

*Riboflavin, vitamin $B_2$*   Riboflavin is found in most of the same foods as thiamin and is more versatile. Rather than being a coenzyme, it is blended by the body with other micronutrients and chemicals to form several enzymes which break down carbohydrates, fats, and proteins into useful forms. It also appears to be extremely important to the skin and similar membranes since its shortages are associated with disorders in those areas. It is destroyed by alcohol and its deficiency is often a severe problem for alcoholics.

*Niacin, vitamin $B_3$*   Niacin (a derivative of the poison nicotine) is the third B vitamin that is both found in and is essential for the digestion of foods containing carbohydrates. It works with its brothers, thiamin and riboflavin, to convert carbohydrates into usable forms, acting to form enzymes, like riboflavin, rather than activating them as does thiamin. Since the body can convert one of the essential amino acids into niacin, it is more rarely deficient than the previous two. It also is part of a coenzyme that aids in skin functions. The disease associated with niacin deficiency is called pellagra, which combines gastrointestinal disorders with the skin problems.

Niacin is found in greater quantities in foods rich in the particular amino acid to which it is related, especially milk and eggs, than its relatives, as well as in red meat and poultry, plus such vegetables as peas, beans, and nuts that contain all the essential amino acids. Strict vegetarians, therefore, are more subject to niacin deficiencies than those of the other vitamins.

*Pyridoxine, vitamin $B_6$*  Vitamin $B_6$ is another very versatile vitamin, being a key coenzyme in the digestion of proteins and in a whole spectrum of conversions of one amino acid to another, as well as in the creation of niacin from its protein source. It is also essential in converting stored glycogen into glucose. Obviously, it is very important in an athlete's diet. Protein diets require a great deal more $B_6$ than do diets high in carbohydrates, the metabolism of which relies more on thiamin, riboflavin, and niacin. Liver, avocados, peas, beans, and nuts, as well as whole grains, yeast, sweet potatoes, bananas, and molasses are all good sources of pyridoxine (whose fiery name indicates its relation to coal tar).

Animal proteins are not high in $B_6$, but when eaten in large quantities will provide a reasonable amount, except for diets with a high percentage of protein (since then they will use up more than they give). The shortage of any of these vitamins that assist digestion does not mean that you will incur deficiency-related diseases. The shortage signals a reduced ability to effectively assimilate the nutritious elements of the food, rendering some of the carbohydrates, fats, and proteins nutritionally useless.

*Cobalamin, vitamin $B_{12}$*  Vitamin $B_{12}$ is identified with creating a balance in the blood system. It is stored in the body for long periods of time and is otherwise only found in animal foods, including milk. Its aid in developing blood cells may be the basis for its fame as an anti-stress cure, since it helps anemia sufferers. It derives its name from being the only vitamin that includes the rare element cobalt. It is also believed to assist in the synthesis of DNA and to aid in the smooth functioning of the nervous system. As with $B_6$, vegetarians risk deficiency, but much more so with $B_{12}$ since it is not found at all in vegetables or fruit.

*Biotin*  The remaining B vitamins have not been graced with a number but still perform important roles. Biotin, which is made in the body by intestinal bacteria and is also found in organ meats and green vegetables, acts as a coenzyme in the formation of fatty acids. It also seems to play a significant role in other

42

digestive functions. The body needs only minute quantities and therefore deficiencies are rare.

*Choline* Choline is one of the disputed vitamins. The U.S. government has not provided a Recommended Daily Allowance but many authorities consider it to be a true vitamin along with inositol, PABA and vitamin P, also known as citrin. Choline (whose name comes from the Greek word for bile) appears to play an important role in the metabolism of fat. In addition, it is one of the components, along with inositol, of lecithin, which is a natural product of the liver and is found in certain animal foods, particularly eggs. Lecithin is an emulsifier; it prevents fat globules from forming and breaks down existing ones. Many health authorities believe that lecithin plays a key role in reducing fat deposits in the bloodstream.

Choline is another vitamin that the body can produce from amino acids. It is also found in calf's liver, peas and beans, dark leafy vegetables, whole grain wheat, and yeast.

*Folic Acid* There is no dispute about the bona fides of folic acid. It is a key assistant to other vitamins, including $B_{12}$, and it is important in the production of red blood cells. It also appears to play a major role in synthesizing DNA and RNA, the key genetic transmitters. Once again, liver and dark green leafy vegetables (from which it gets its name), along with whole wheat, are important sources, as are yeast, chicken, and salmon. The body can store it, so its daily dietary needs are not as essential, and it can be produced in the intestinal tract as well. It appears to be extremely important to pregnant women.

*Inositol* The controversial inositol, the other constituent with choline in the body's production of lecithin, has been the beneficiary of a variety of claims including that when combined with certain other of the B vitamins it will help retard hair loss and even regenerate hair. Oranges, grapefruit, watermelon, and other melons along with peas, beans, liver, and oysters are good sources of inositol, whose name indicates that it is an alcohol that gives strength.

*Pantothenic Acid*  Another B vitamin that is important in the body's assimilation of carbohydrates, fats, and protein, pantothenic acid also works as a coenzyme. Found throughout the body (whence its name), it is believed to help the adrenal glands as well as aid the proper functioning of the nervous system and the production of certain hormones. It is found in most of the same foods as its brethren $B_1$, $B_2$, and $B_3$.

*Para-Aminobenzoic Acid (PABA)*  PABA, on the other hand, does not share the same reviews on all sides as its almost equally unpronounceable cousin, pantothenic acid. PABA recently acquired popularity as an aid against sunburn, and is found in many high Sun Protection Factor sunscreens. It helps the body form folic acid and its deficiency may cause skin problems as well as graying hair. Once again, it tends to be found in the typical B vitamin foods.


## VITAMIN C

No vitamin has a more historically clear value or controversial present-day claims than vitamin C. Over two hundred years ago the British discovered that certain citrus fruit could cure scurvy among the sailors at sea. In fact, their use of limes on board has come down to haunt them as a nickname. Vitamin C, also known as ascorbic acid for its a[nti] scorbute (or scurvy) properties, is still best found in oranges, grapefruit, and the other citrus fruit, though it is also found in most other fruit (including tomatoes) in lesser concentrations, as well as potatoes and green vegetables, especially green peppers. It is necessary to maintain vitamin C in the diet since the body eliminates it when not immediately used.

Aside from averting scurvy, it is known to aid in the formation of collagen, one of two proteins (the other being elastin) essential to healthy, flexible skin, and in keeping cell walls throughout the body from breaking down. These qualities may result from its anti-oxidizing properties, for which vitamin E is better known. Starting with Nobel Laureate Linus Pauling's advocacy, vitamin C has also been viewed as, if not a cure for, at least an important aid in overcoming the common cold. It is also considered by many to assist in battling cancers and in fighting infections of all kinds.

## VITAMIN D

What vitamin A is to eyes, vitamin D is to bones and teeth. It plays its role by assisting the body to absorb calcium and phosphorus more efficiently. That is why excessive doses can result in calcium deposits and overly brittle bones. Chemically, vitamin D is a derivative of cholesterol. Ultra-violet radiation, usually from sunlight, photosynthesizes the basic chemical structure of vitamin D all over human skin. However, people who, due to climatic or other reasons, do not expose significant skin to sunlight may not produce enough vitamin D internally. Its most common external sources are fortified milk, although fish with an oily texture to their flesh, like tuna, salmon, and mackerel, and egg yolk also provide significant vitamin D. And, as with vitamin A, the historic nostrum of our elders, cod liver oil, may well be the best single source.

## VITAMIN E

At first dismissed by orthodox health specialists as a fad, vitamin E has now been generally accepted as one of the most important parts of our diet. While claims for its ability to bolster one's sex life and reduce the risk of coronary disease remain unsubstantiated, the ability of vitamin E to oppose the attack by oxygen on various chemical substances is now wholly accepted. This has at least one clearly beneficial effect, protecting fats and vitamins that are fat soluble, like vitamin A, from being broken down in the system. A popular theory is that this oxygenation of fatty substances causes the eventual hardening and drying out of the cells and is at the heart of aging. Oxygen's attack is led by substances called "free radicals," which are believed to be opposed by vitamin E.

Its claims for being an aphrodisiac relate to the effects of vitamin E deficiencies on animals in certain experiments. Muscular degeneration, particularly of those involved in reproduction, has been found in animals with vitamin E deficiencies. In fact, the generic name for the four types of vitamin E, tocopherol, is from the Greek for bringing about childbirth. For the athlete, the potential value of vitamin E lies in its alleged ability to assist cardiovascular functions, its partially proven ability to protect skin surfaces, especially those in the lungs, from oxidizing pollutants, and its established role in keeping muscle tissue from being broken down by oxygen molecules and enabling the body to better use its oxygen intake. The latter function appears to be most important when exercising in the relatively oxygen-poor atmosphere at high altitudes.

The best sources of vitamin E are vegetable oils and fresh wheat germ. Red meat and green leafy vegetables along with carrots and eggs are also good. When vitamin E is found in supplements, the most commonly used formula is the one that is also most common in nature, alpha tocopherol. But as noted above, there are actually four kinds and it is believed that at least one of the other three is a more effective anti-oxident than alpha. Therefore a supplement that provides all four in a mixture should be superior.

## VITAMIN K

Vitamin K has been established to be essential in the clotting of the blood which prevents hemorrhaging. Since it is found in most vegetables and cereals, and is produced in additional quantities inside the intestine (except in newborns who lack the proper bacteria), deficiencies are rare. However, if you are taking antibiotics or sulfa drugs for a long period of time, which kill off the bacteria, a supplement may be needed. It is obviously most needed by athletes engaged in activities like boxing in which minor cuts are a frequent companion.

## VITAMIN P

Another "maybe" vitamin is citrin, known as vitamin P, for permeability. It may be essential for maintaining the integrity of capillary walls to withstand unwanted breakdowns from cell to cell. It may also assist vitamin C in maintaining the flexibility of collagen throughout skin tissue. As its popular name suggests, it is found largely in connection with citrus fruit, mostly in the pulp and inside the peel. In health food stores and vitamin supplements it is often included under the rubric "Bioflavonoids."

## VITAMIN SUPPLEMENTS

The major dispute over vitamins is which, if any, should be taken in supplement form, and then in what dosages. However, there is also disagreement over whether or not wholly synthetic vitamins perform the same function as those in nature. It is axiomatic that the chemical compounds in the body cannot distinguish the source of another chemical compound. The proponents of natural vitamins argue that when taken in food or in a slightly impure natural form, vitamins come with enzymes or minerals or other nutrients that lead to better and more complete use by the body of the original vitamins. For example, nature packages its B complex vitamins with carbohydrates. In either case, as long as megadoses are not being taken (since in some cases megadoses can be toxic to certain people), the placebo effect will rule; if you believe in it, it will help you no matter what. Since between natural and synthetic you can't really lose, it's only a question of getting the right amount of bang per buck.

# Minerals

Like vitamins, there is no question that certain amounts of specific minerals are essential for good health. Also, like vitamins, there are great disputes over which ones are necessary for what and in which dosages. Clearly, sodium and chloride, which make up salt, calcium, potassium, iron, iodine, and phosphorus are necessary because of their prevalence in cells, bones, and enzymes. Also, magnesium, zinc, and copper serve many functions. Others also appear in minute quantities, some with clearly proven uses, like molybdenum, which is part of a key enzyme, and some, like selenium, which are believed to have uses, in this case perhaps assisting vitamin E.

## CALCIUM AND PHOSPHORUS

These two minerals are the building blocks of the skeletal system. Calcium, above all, is essential to strong t 'th and bones. Surprisingly, it makes up only about 2 percent of the average person's total weight. Human bones are basically porous. The most common source of dietary calcium is milk and milk products, but it is also found in green leafy vegetables, citrus fruit, and some peas and beans.

The way calcium combines with phosphorus is both boon and bust, since the two work together, but are needed in balance. While phosphorus is also in milk, plus other sources of complete protein, too often processed foods contain phosphates but not enough calcium. Some offenders are frequent parts of the diet, like carbonated soft drinks. As a result, a relative deficiency of calcium can occur, which can lead to the same problems of bone weakness and stunted growth.

## IRON

Another famous mineral that is properly associated with its real bodily need is iron. It helps the blood carry oxygen from the lungs to all the cells to perform the chemical reactions needed to produce the energy that heats and moves the body. Iron is a tricky devil, since it is only absorbed into the system when various other elements are present. That is why it, along with certain other minerals, is sometimes put in supplements in a chelated form, one that has been altered by a process designed to reflect how the body treats them so that they can be more fully used. In the nonchelated form which is found naturally (and from cooking with iron pots), it needs to be associated with an acid to be absorbed and the presence of calcium also appears to be important. Foods that are high in iron include red meat, fish, and poultry, as well as green leafy vegetables, like Popeye's spinach. An interesting aspect of the need for acid, and possibly vitamin C, is that two American classics may well provide the right combinations for iron—beef and potatoes and orange juice plus an iron-enriched cereal.

An athlete's need for iron is obvious. To meet the greater demands of muscles for oxygen, caused by increased exertion, the iron must be present. A shortage of iron can result in a weakened condition from anemia and a strange craving to watch Geritol commercials.


## IODINE

Eating the filings from an iron bar is one thing, but quaffing iodine is quite another. Nevertheless, it is no less essential to proper health than the other minerals or any vitamin. It plays its key role in the thyroid gland, stimulating the production of the thyroxine hormone which regulates metabolism and the rate of production and use of energy. While the thyroid appears to play an absolutely critical role during the growth periods of childhood and adolescence, it is by no means vestigial in adulthood. An iodine deficiency may have a direct effect on production of thyroxine which will in turn lower the metabolic rate and reduce stamina and energy. There are relatively few food sources of iodine in nature, basically seafood and saltwater fish and such oriental cooking items as kelp and other seaweed. The most universal source of iodine is iodized salt.


## POTASSIUM AND SODIUM

These two relatively common dietary minerals are "Mr. Inside" and "Mr. Outside" in our cells. Potassium is found in the fluid inside the cell walls while sodium is found almost exclusively in the fluids that surround the cells. They are believed to create the chemical balance to allow transmission of the electrical impulses that control and receive commands from the neurological system. That is why they are often called electrolytes. The key role they play in maintaining balanced fluid levels and pressures shows up in the relatively quick deficiency symptoms, starting with thirst. As far as athletes are concerned though, the most significant early deficiencies cause muscle cramping.

The two minerals must maintain the balance which is necessary to allow the nutrients and essential parts of our cellular and tissue structures to flow freely. While perspiration does deplete sodium, it mostly depletes water, and not potassium. Many specialists now recommend that salt tablets should only be reserved for excessively long exercise in very hot weather and only after a great deal of plain water has been used to try to maintain the liquid balance. On the other hand, when salt is taken it ought to be in conjunction with potassium rich sources. An excellent way to do that is with orange juice. Bananas are also a classic source of potassium, which is also found in meat, peas, beans, whole grains, potatoes, and, interestingly, coffee and tea. Sodium, of course, is in salt plus all seafood and saltwater fish. All too frequently, it is also found in a snow-like covering applied from a little white shaker whose natural habitat is the American table. This excess throws the body's balance completely out of kilter, and is considered to be a leading source of high blood pressure (hypertension) related to the extra work the heart and cardiovascular system must perform when the body retains water in the system to try to maintain the desired salinity levels. Obviously, an excess of sodium punishes an athlete by requiring every muscle to work in a sponge-like environment.


## CHLORINE

Sodium's companion in salt, chlorine, also is an important part of cellular fluids but is most essential for its role in creating, with hydrogen, hydrochloric acid, the primary actor in breaking down food in the stomach. Chlorine also acts in the lymphatic system and throughout the body in much the same way that it does in the swimming pool, by cleaning out the waste (through stimulating the liver). Of course, most sources of sodium are also sources of chlorine since it is part of salt, though it is found in many leafy greens as well.


## COPPER, MAGNESIUM, AND ZINC

These three classy metals are examples of the elements found in minute quantities that most people would never conceive of as being essential to good health. Nevertheless, magnesium plays almost as important a role in bone structure as do calcium and phosphorus, magnesium being very similar in properties to phosphorus. Copper helps in the formation of red blood cells and is believed to be one of the elements that must be present for iron to be properly utilized by the body. Zinc is the most versatile of all, playing a role in an enormous variety of enzymes. Zinc also has a strong relationship in the minds of many nutritionists and biologists to healthy reproductive organs.

Shortages of magnesium create muscular weaknesses and cramping, similar to those caused by deficiencies of potassium or sodium. Copper deficiencies tend to be blood related, as well as causing problems with the lungs, since they seem to be involved with respiratory enzymes. Zinc may be an unimportant deficiency on the playing field, since it is blamed for failures in the reproductive area, but it certainly might be important in keeping an athlete in a proper frame of mind. Magnesium is found in green leafy vegetables, oil-rich nuts and seeds, whole grains, and egg yolk. Copper and zinc are found mainly in liver and other organ meats as well as oysters (perhaps rightly known for their sexual powers) and certain whole grains. Milk is also a good source of zinc.


# Supplementary Supplements

Nowhere is the concept that one person's panacea is another's placebo more obvious than in discussions of supplements other than vitamins and minerals. An example that is popular with some athletes and many other health fans is bee pollen, touted by its users as a perfect nutrition source, high in vitamins, minerals, and enzymes. Orthodox nutritionists scoff at the thought that in the dosage levels that are usually consumed the amount of nutrients involved could be helpful. What is clear is that bee pollen is a natural product of intense protein, vitamin, and mineral content. Whether or not it provides satisfactory quantities to be useful is another question. It certainly does not appear to be harmful in any way.

# Fluids

There is one other essential food—water. We are all more sponge than steel. But it is more complicated then just filling 'er up. Water is our universal solvent and it is moved around by the body to dissolve concentrations of any substance that is above the desired levels. Therefore it is attracted to sugar and salt in the stomach, causing a shortage elsewhere. Since it is the missing link between glycogen and glucose, its rushing to the stomach can leave an energy gap in the muscles. Balance is the key. Just as the sodium/potassium ratio must be right for proper utilization of nutrients at the cell level, dilution of hydrochloric acid in the stomach, or too much or too little moisture in the rest of the digestive tract, can cause incomplete digestion or cramps. The drinking of sugared or high sodium or potassium liquids can upset both the cellular and digestive fluid balances. That's why drinking anything except straight water to quench thirst during and after exercise should be done only in moderation, or dilution.

# A Case History

Great athletes develop their dietary regimes around the aforementioned principles, and trial and error. A perfect example of this is a man who has had tremendous success in competition over many years, and even greater popularity. **Arnold Palmer** almost single-handedly made professional golf a major American attraction through the patented closing rushes that created and galvanized Arnie's Army. And while golf does not bring to mind the kind of strenuous exertion required of other competitive sports, Palmer still walks an average of five to six miles per round and runs three miles a day on his own. His popularity has created an additional drain for him. Just getting from his car to the clubhouse signing autographs all the way can be quite an exercise.

Palmer's diet is very sensible and modified for his sport. A believer in flushing out the system, he starts the day with a full pitcher of water with the juice of one lemon squeezed into it. A bit later his breakfast will be fresh fruit juice, a boiled egg with bacon and a piece of buttered whole wheat toast. This is his main fuel for the day, a good mix which includes quick energy fructose from the juice, slow burning carbohydrates in the toast, fats in the bacon and the butter, protein from the egg and bacon, and a mixture of micronutrients, nutrients needed only in microscopic quantities, throughout. Lunch during a match is something like half a chicken sandwich—again slow burning and low calorie. In fact, Palmer recently lost some weight by cutting down on red meat and eating more fish and chicken.

Around the sixteenth hole, Palmer retrieves the snack his wife Winnie provides him. She knows that he is so wrapped up in the match that on his own he would forget to eat entirely, so she makes sure he has something like granola bars along for a burst of extra endurance over the last three holes. Following a day on the links, Palmer tries to avoid going to bed with a stomach full of sleep-impeding heavy foods by both eating as early as possible and focussing on lighter courses. Baked or broiled fish and roast chicken are his leading candidates, never anything fried, and nothing like potatoes with heavy gravy. He also limits his alcohol to beer.

Besides a light, balanced diet, Palmer adds the need for sleep as a must. "Sleep replaces my energy," he feels. So it's early to bed, around 10:00 P.M., and early to rise, about 5:30 A.M. (and off to jog). On top of this good regimen, he takes a multiple vitamin supplement daily along with alfalfa tablets (a traditional herbal-ist treatment for arthritis) to help alleviate any aches or pains from the day before.

Palmer shows us that anyone who wants to stay physically active has to pay attention to his or her diet and lifestyle. His regime is hard to argue with, unless you're allergic to alfalfa. But it also is suited to a sport that requires calm concentration and mental and physical stamina over a four-day tournament. Over the next ten chapters we'll hear from other superstars in a wide variety of strenuous sports. The goal is to match your lifestyle to what makes sense for you, taking their advice and applying it to your needs.

# CHAPTER THREE

# Baseball

With 162 games in the regular season alone and few days off, baseball requires an endurance and pacing that are not needed for any other sport. However, baseball is popularly identified with all the wrong foods—from the hot dogs, soda, and beer sold at most ballparks to the crackerjack stanza of "Take Me Out to the Ball Game" to candy bars made famous by Babe Ruth and Reggie Jackson. Nor is there a training table tradition to regiment the players. Nevertheless, some of the top stars of the game and their trainers are extremely conscious of their dietary needs. Even someone as apparently carefree and full of *joie de vivre* as **Reggie Jackson** curbs his spontaneity in favor of a planned diet. He, for example, avoids red meat and will only eat a large brunch (usually scrambled eggs with bacon or sausages plus cold cereal) before night games. After the game, it's a light dinner, preferably fish (his favorite is swordfish) or chicken.

One generality that seems to hold true to baseball is that because of batting and fielding practice, no one gets to eat normally before a day game (so when a player refers to eating before or after a game, it means the now more common night games). Also, starting pitchers tend to adjust their diet to the team's pitching rotation and older players who remain in the game are more serious about their diets than rookies. The other general point to remember is that baseball draws from a great variety of cultures in the Western Hemisphere. That means that Mexico's export to the Dodgers, Fernando Valenzuela, and Campy

Campaneris, Cuba's gift to several teams, to name just two of many, may thrive before a game on spicy Latin dishes that would do in a Steve Garvey or Robin Yount. And a good ol' Southern boy like Dale Murphy, the Atlanta Braves' slugging centerfielder (and the National League's 1982 and 1983 MVP), whose dietary philosophy to keep his weight up is "Eat anything that doesn't move," can get away with heaps of country cooking that would slow down a Northerner like big Dave Winfield.

Because of the long season, professional baseball players play as many away games as there are both home and away games in the entire season of hockey and basketball, the sports with the next greatest number of games. That means a lot of time spent in hotels (especially on rainy days), airports, and airplanes. As anyone who has traveled the pathways of America knows, it is much easier to find a processed-cheese-food meat-by-product burger than a good broiled chicken and a fresh salad with pure virgin olive oil dressing. The allure of fast food parlors and the $32.50 a day allowance for meal money that burns in their pockets combine to wreak havoc with all but the most stalwart diet devotees. (Up from eight dollars in 1961, the $32.50 is known as "Murphy Money" in honor of former pitcher Johnny Murphy, whose accomplishment as player rep in the tranquil prestrike days B.M.M. (Before Marvin Miller) was to fatten this allotment.)

It is against this backdrop that Major League baseball players must function, eight months a year, seven days a week. This is how they do it, followed by some favorite recipes and a dietary scheme proposed by Jim Warfield, trainer for the Cleveland Indians and Gene Monahan, trainer of the N.Y. Yankees.

# Heavy Hitters:
## First Basemen and Outfielders

Long time All-Star first baseman for the Dodgers, now with the San Diego Padres, thirty-six year old **Steve Garvey** has converted his strong feelings about nutrition into the all-time National League record for consecutive game appearances (more than twelve hundred games nonstop over ten years). All-American good looks and Popeye forearms are his hallmarks. Garvey feels that the proper diet, rest, and a daily exercise program are the three essential ingredients for looking well and feeling fit. He credits this combination for the stamina that enabled him to establish the NL iron-man record.

During the season, Garvey believes in eating carbohydrates, but stays away from refined and highly processed foods. Only occasionally will he give in and have a Big Mac. When he travels he depends on a few good restaurants in each city that he knows prepare some special dishes, or their regular dishes just the way he likes them. He avoids eating for five hours before a game and rarely uses salt. Breakfast on a game day consists of pancakes and fruit, his favorite being melon, usually cantaloupe or honeydew, with fresh orange or grapefruit juice. If he's not playing that day, he will eat two eggs, cold bran cereal and tea with lemon. If he eats bread, it is only rye, pumpernickel or whole wheat, never white. Lunch is normally his biggest meal, and he will have something rich in protein—generally seafood, swordfish or halibut, chicken or veal. "Once a week I will eat beef for energy, but I try to stay away from it as much as possible. Because of this, I feel my lipids and triglycerides have gone down considerably." Dinner is generally a salad, a small portion of chicken or fish, and vegetables, especially the dark green leafy ones such as spinach. After a game he eats lightly, so as not to go to bed with a full stomach. And just to play it safe, he takes at least five thousand milligrams of vitamin C plus a multiple and B complex vitamins.

For those who always said Garvey can't possibly be as perfect as everyone thinks, here is some good news. "My weakness is dessert," he admits. "I can never pass them up, although I try to stay away from them as much as possible. Instead, I will have fresh fruit salads, perhaps a mixture of apples, pears, and something exotic like kiwi."

Steve's heavy bat was needed in San Diego to plug the large hole left when **Dave Winfield** moved East to the Yankees. At a towering six feet, six inches, Winfield is one of the most feared batters in baseball—and also one of the nicest guys. He always seems to have time for his favorite charities (especially the Dave Winfield Foundation which he set up). In fact, the day I interviewed him, he stopped on his way from the dugout to the locker room not only to autograph a baseball for a handicapped young man but also to give him the cap he was wearing. Of course, pitchers don't get to see that side of him. One of the few players who has punished opposing batteries in both leagues, he is also a graceful Golden Glove fielder, who led all Major League outfielders in 1982 with seventeen assists. Whether his prowess is only because he chews on sunflower seeds instead of tobacco during the game is unknown, however. He also eschews red meat entirely and eats only fish and fowl. Winfield finds that he gets all the power he needs from his usual chef salad lunch made from cheese, turkey, and all kinds of mixed greens (but no ham).

He avoids big dinners after the game, agreeing with the theory that since you need fewer calories when you are asleep, going to bed with food in your digestive tract can only make you fat. Winfield takes no vitamin supplements but gets a boost from the sunflower seeds (which are high in protein and calories and rich in minerals including zinc). Says Big Dave: "A good tip for younger ball players is to buy whole sunflower seeds instead of chewing tobacco. The process of popping them in your mouth, opening them, taking out the seeds, then spitting out the shells and chewing the seeds is easily as relaxing and obviously much healthier than chewing either gum or tobacco."

**Pete Rose,** or Charley Hustle as he is known to his fans, has won championships in both Cincinnati and Philadelphia and is now the best-known player in Canada, starring with the Montreal Expos. He leads all active players in the Majors in virtually every lifetime offensive category (except HRs and RBIs). His reckless style of play gives no hint of the importance he gives to his diet. While careening head first into bases might not sound like the best plan for longevity, Rose takes a lot better care of himself when dealing with plates other than home.

"Nutrition," he believes, "is extremely important in the life of an athlete, and if you eat the right foods you don't even have to take vitamins. The most essential point is to have a good meal to start off the day." Rose eats only two meals a day both on and off season, but it is the one in the morning that sets him up for the rest of the day. For night games, he arises late and has a substantial brunch before going to the ball park. This consists of soup and broiled fish or steak. He won't eat again until after the game and then it will only be a light sandwich. When Rose plays a day game he has a large breakfast: eggs, fresh orange juice, fruit, and coffee, which he limits to one cup a day. He will then have a big dinner—chicken or fish, vegetables, and a salad. His favorite drink is ice tea and he highly recommends substituting fresh juices for sodas. His sound advice: "Cut all sweets out of your diet and never skip the first meal of the day." Considering that Rose has been on base more than anyone else in the sport's history, he must be doing something right.

Rookie of the Year in 1967, Most Valuable Player ten years later, the Joe Cronin Award for Distinguished Achievement in 1975, and more Batting Championships than anyone since Ty Cobb (1969, 1972, 1973, 1974, 1975, 1977, and 1978 to be exact) —there is absolutely no question about who is the best batsman in baseball. **Rod Carew,** with a lifetime average over .330, is strictly in a class by himself when it comes to stroking base hits. Though now the first baseman for the California Angels, he was also a standout second baseman for the Minnesota Twins, at which position he established records of hits, triples, average and stolen bases (and is second or third in virtually all other lifetime batting categories).

His tastes at the table have one thing in common with his hitting—it goes to all fields. On game days, Carew believes in getting in two meals before going to the ball park. He starts the day with a bowl of cold cereal, usually Wheaties or Corn Flakes, with a glass of milk, or he will have a ham and cheese omelette with a glass of fresh orange juice. He is also a vitamin devotee, taking a multiple every day plus extra B complex and calcium when he feels tired. Lunch is lemonade and either a bacon, lettuce, and tomato or club sandwich, or a small hamburger. He won't eat anything then until after the game. If he's on the road, he'll usually have fish (preferably trout), a salad, and a glass of wine to relax. When he's home, Carew's wife will make him macaroni and cheese or his favorite, hot dogs and beans (Carew describes the way she cuts up the hot dogs and mixes them with the beans with such total relish that it almost makes you believe that it has to be good for you). "I like pies and desserts but I try not to have them. I'm not that big an eater in any case. In fact, off-season I usually skip lunch entirely. On the other hand, that is when I eat the pies and ice cream that I can't afford to eat when I'm playing." His favorite food of all is the Szechuan cuisine of Northern China. "I'll go out to dinner and order three or four different dishes at one sitting—hot spicy beef, chicken with cashews, and shrimp or lobster with rice are the ones I like the best." That's appropriate, since Carew is one guy who could bat .300 even using chopsticks.

The two most impressive single season Major League marks set in 1982 were by the same man, **Rickey Henderson.** The Oakland A's flash is in the record books with the dubious distinction of most times caught stealing (42). But to dispel any idea that his on-base appearances warmed the hearts of pitchers and catchers, his other record was the incredibly felonious 130 times he successfully filched an extra ninety feet around the diamond, a category in which he also led the majors in 1983 (with a paltry 108). He unsettled his opponents so much, that Henderson also led the Majors in 1982 in walks with 116. That made 246 total bases without the need to hit the ball. Not surprisingly, he was named the 1982 recipient of the Joe Cronin Award for Distinguished Achievement.

To stay light on his feet, Henderson keeps his diet light too. "My mother always used to say I had such a little stomach. In fact, the circumference of my legs is as big as my waist. I don't really care too much about food. If I don't like what people are serving, I just go without dinner." But at five feet, ten inches and 185 pounds, Henderson does have very specific ideas about how to maintain his energy and physique. "I always have a big breakfast. This consists of bacon and eggs, grits, a large piece of melon, and a large glass of fresh orange juice. I like light lunches, usually a big salad, sometimes broiled seafood, and sometimes a hamburger and a milkshake. After batting practice I'll take an orange for energy. It's after the game that I like to eat. Then it will be a steak or fish or chicken with a baked potato and vegetables, my favorite being a mixture of sweet peas, carrots, and corn. If I eat bread, it's whole wheat, and although I don't believe in carbohydrate loading, I sometimes eat spaghetti. For dessert I like fresh fruit pies (especially blueberry) with ice cream on top. My only other rules are that I don't drink, just an occasional glass of wine, and I take a multivitamin supplement every day."

A clue to Henderson's metabolism is his disclosure that while some players like to relax on a game day, he likes to get "hyper." To balance this he feels he needs nine or ten hours of sleep a night to keep in top form. Altogether the picture is very much one of a high energy, high octane machine.

Unlike Henderson, **Lou Piniella,** the AL Rookie of the Year back in 1969, and the Yankees ageless hitting maestro (1982's leading Designated Hitter at .344 and the number two pinch hitter at .360), does not earn his keep or stats with his speed. In fact, his career stolen base totals are about one hundred below Rickey's 1982 production. Nevertheless, when Lou reported for spring training a few seasons ago over his preferred playing weight, Yankee principal owner George Steinbrenner ordered him to lose it—at least eight pounds. The fine was more severe than the diet. "The hardest part," admits Piniella, "was leaving the table hungry and giving up the things I like—soft drinks, beer, butter, bread." The diet was a quick weight loss program that he used to take the weight off and that he returns to every time the weight creeps back on. It consists of a breakfast of half a grapefruit or grapefruit juice, lunch of soup and fruit, and dinner of a small piece of fish or chicken and a green vegetable.

# Mounds of Talent:
# Pitchers

From his first year in the Bigs (NL Rookie of the Year in 1967), it was obvious that if he stayed healthy **Tom Seaver** was a Hall of Famer. Three Cy Young Awards, three E.R.A. lead-erships, two National League Championships, and one Ama-zin' World Series victory with the Mets later, Seaver's ticket to Cooperstown is safe. Always a thinking man's pitcher, he is also very thoughtful about his diet. "The secret to playing well and feeling fit is to eat a balanced diet, to stay away from all junk foods and to substitute things that are good for you. Candy, cakes, etc., can be replaced by fruit, and empty calories should give way to vegetables and salads. Breakfast is usually poached eggs on dry whole grain toast with either grapefruit or cantaloupe, depending on what's in season. Or I'll just have cold cereal, Raisin Bran or Wheaties. If I'm pitching, lunch is at one o'clock for an evening game. Then it will be cold chicken or a tunafish or steak sandwich with fresh fruit salad and some cottage cheese. After the game, I don't eat much, just a light dinner because it's late. A very good lunch, one I often have on the road, is a chef salad. When they are well made, they include greens for roughage and vegetables for vitamins and minerals, all mixed in with protein such as cheese and turkey. I will have a steak every once in a while, but most of the time I try to stay away from red meat and eat fish or chicken instead." Tom's belief in balance and moderation keeps his diet in perspective. For example, he drinks beer occa-sionally and likes wine. "My weakness is ice cream and home-made cookies, but in general I try not to have too many sweets." And as National Leaguers know, what Seaver tries to do, he almost always accomplishes.

One of Steve Garvey's San Diego teammates who is also serious about nutrition is **Eric Show,** the Padres' young pitch-ing sensation. He has found that eating a variety of wholesome and nutritious foods, including plenty of vegetables, and avoid-ing caffeine, junk food and excess dietary fat have given him a lot more energy. While he feels that he is still learning about nutrition, as a physics major at the University of California in Riverside (his hometown), he knows something about energy. However, Show is trying to combine the two disciplines. In jargon atypical of dugout banter, he explains his ideas about Zen theory, how the electromagnetic fields of the body interfere with the nerve functions and how nutrition relates to all this and the maintenance of a proper chi energy flow. Whew!

As to more mundane matters, on the nights before he pitches, Show insists on at least ten hours of sleep and he tries to get at least eight hours on his off days. He feels much better having given up junk food, although a while back he quit sugar cold turkey and became sick. Sugar, he now feels, is necessary to digest protein, and whether it be fructose or glucose, all sugars are basically the same. Honey is probably the best, according to Show, as it is much less processed than plain white sugar and contains minerals. He also believes that less is more, so at home he tries not to have too many desserts, soda, or candy. If he needs the energy of simple carbohydrates, he'll go straight to some honey.

He takes a multi-vitamin each day and starts with a solid breakfast: eggs (but no greasy sausages), ham and potatoes, whole wheat toast and tea or, if he's not that hungry, just a plain omelette. Lunch is usually limited to one ham and cheese or steak sandwich, as he doesn't like to eat a lot on the day of a game. Dinner after the game is usually substantial. He'll have a juicy steak, salad, and potatoes with tea or water. He doesn't drink hard liquor or wine but will occasionally quaff a beer. On the days that he pitches, which are generally one out of every five, he will not eat heavily. "The blood that is needed for digestion can best be used on other things—like my pitching arm," he contends. Although Show is a firm believer in good nutrition and exercise (off-season he runs a couple of miles every day and lifts weights), he does have one encouraging thing to say to people who depress easily on this subject: "Much of it is genetic."

Someone who easily depresses opposing batters is his new teammate **Rich "Goose" Gossage,** probably the most awesome pitcher in baseball today. In baseball parlance, the Goose throws BBs. His effect on batters is reminiscent of Lefty Gomez's famous story about batting against Bob Feller in a thick fog. The home plate umpire asked why he lit a match and held it in front of his nose, suggesting that it wouldn't help him see Feller's blazing fastballs. Gomez's response was: "I just want to make sure he sees *me*." Goose's glowering six foot, five inch mustachioed presence gives no hint of his more delicate eating habits: he actually loves salads and small sandwiches.

While not exactly a health nut, he has a basically well-planned diet. Breakfast at home is usually orange juice plus eggs and bacon, or Raisin Bran. If he might be pitching that night, he will have an early lunch consisting of either pork chops or chicken, and a green salad. On his salad, he will have ranch style dressing. After that he won't eat anything until after the game. Then he will have whatever is in the clubhouse, but he keeps it light. Chinese food is his favorite and whenever he can, Goose goes for his ideal dinner—chop suey; a mixture of Chinese vegetables including water chestnuts, mushrooms, and peppers. If he gets home around 11:30 P.M. after a game, and hasn't eaten, he will then have a tuna sandwich. In any case, he does not eat desserts, and tries to stay away from sugar entirely because he feels it is just empty calories.

Since Goose may pitch three or four days in a row and then not again for a week, he can't afford jetlag. His solution is to have a big breakfast. "I'm never on any kind of schedule," he admits. "But when I get up, if I eat a large meal it will set me up for the rest of the day and my body will automatically adjust to the right time schedule."

Like Eric Show, the Houston Astros' ace **Nolan Ryan** pitches for a club just up the road from his hometown, and like Gossage, he throws "smoke." In 1983, Ryan broke the fifty-six-year-old Major League career strike-out record of Walter "Big Train" Johnson, 3,509 Ks, and is now locked in a battle with Steve Carlton to push the all-time level ever upward. A true superstar in both leagues and on both coasts (having pitched in both New York for the Mets and California for the Angels), Ryan nevertheless has his feet firmly on the ground when it comes to nutrition: "Athletes are no different than the general public; what is good for them is good for everyone. The general rules are to stay away from excess sugars, white starches (bread, cakes, etc.), and additional salt

64

(other than what is found in food naturally). The same goes for vitamin supplements. If you eat right, you don't need them."

For breakfast he eats half a cantaloupe or a half grape-fruit, a bowl of cold cereal, usually Raisin Bran, with fruit, bananas or peaches cut up in it, and a slice of whole grain toast. Lunch is a well-balanced mixture of salad, meat, chicken or fish, and fresh vegetables. After the game, he'll eat something light like another bowl of cereal or a sandwich. If he's not playing, he will have chopped steak or a chicken dish.

Ryan believes that meat has essential vitamins that one needs as an athlete. "It is food for strength, you need that extra fat for energy. Besides, the chickens today have just as many if not more hormones." But unlike many other nutritionally aware athletes today, he seldom eats pasta. "I'm from a small town in Texas. What did we know about fancy foreign foods like spaghetti? So I never developed a taste for it." By the same logic, what he does like once a week is anything barbe-cued.

The Milwaukee Brewers spell relief *R O L L I E*. And with good reason. In 1981, **Rollie Fingers** became the only reliever to win both the Cy Young and Most Valuable Player awards, capping an unprecedented reign as one of baseball's premier relievers. While most relief pitchers last only a couple of sea-sons, Fingers has been on top since his championship days with the Oakland A's. A fierce competitor, Fingers uses an as-sortment of pitches and artifices to get the job done, the most famous of which was his classic fake intentional walk turned into a key strikeout of Johnny Bench in the 1972 World Series. His diet, however, is much more traditional. At six feet, four inches and 210 pounds, he believes in the basic American sys-tem of protein to keep fit. Fingers starts the day with a bowl of cereal, grapefruit juice, and a cup of coffee. For lunch he has a sandwich—chicken salad or roast beef—or a hamburger. After the game he will have chicken, roast beef, or ham, if he cannot find his favorite food, broiled abalone—not an easy trick in Milwaukee.

# Quicksilver:
# Infielders

The American League's Most Valuable Player in 1982, **Robin Yount** is one of the great young stars of the game. In leading the Milwaukee Brewers to the 1982 American League Championship and one game away from winning the World Series, Yount batted .331 (one point below the major league's highest) and led both Leagues in hits, total bases, and slugging percentage, while also leading the American League in assists by a shortstop. The extent of his athletic skills is indicated by how seriously his teammates and team took the rumors of his foray into professional golf when it looked like, due to an injury, his baseball career would have to be prematurely ended.

At six feet, one inch and 175 pounds, Yount is in excellent shape. He is a firm believer that if you take the proper vitamins (which, in his case, is a single multi-vitamin supplement each day) it doesn't really matter what you eat. Nevertheless, as far as diets go, he follows a pretty good one. Yount doesn't drink alcohol and likes all kinds of vegetables and fruit. His favorite dinners are the complex-carbohydrate-classics spaghetti with meat sauce and macaroni and cheese. For breakfast he has a bowl of cold cereal with a glass of fresh orange juice, and for lunch —cheeseburgers.

Gold Glove third baseman and only the sixth captain of the Yankees, **Graig Nettles** is probably best remembered for his play in the third game of the 1978 World Series against the Dodgers when his brilliant fielding almost single-handedly turned the Series around. At bat, his specialty is round trippers, having led the league in 1976 and being the all-time leading home run hitter among American League third basemen. Never a speed merchant, Nettles lives and dies with his great vision and superior reflexes. It is not surprising that to maintain these he takes vitamin A. Ten thousand units of vitamin A daily along with vitamins E and D plus a multiple is Nettles's program. For energy, he believes in red meat. About two o'clock in the afternoon on a game day, he always tries to have a steak, leaving enough time to digest before going to the ball park. After the game in the evening, all he has is a light snack.

Probably the best pure hitter east of the Rockies is the Kansas City Royals' perennial All-Star, **George Brett.** Elected the American League's Most Valuable Player in 1980, Brett also won his second batting crown that year with an incredible .390 average, the highest in the Majors since Ted Williams's .406 in 1941. Besides learning the art of hitting 'frozen ropes' (baseballese for the kind of stinging line drives that are Brett's specialty) with or without pine tar on the bat, he has tended to watch more closely his calories and intake as he gets older.

During the season Brett rarely eats breakfast; in fact, he will eat only one full size meal, early in the afternoon. He will usually have soup, salad, and fish or chicken. He rarely eats red meat, except for the occasional steak sandwich for lunch. After the game it will be just a light sandwich. Off-season he reverses the process. Lunch will be light, a tuna or egg salad sandwich, while dinner will be the same as his big lunch meal during the season. Brett attributes his love of fish to being raised in California. His two real nonbaseball passions are golf, which is his off-season way to keep his hands, arms, and eyes sharp, and Mexican food, for which he'll forsake his diet and splurge almost anytime, regardless of the effect on his hands, arms, or eyes.

Who's the active National Leaguer with the highest lifetime batting average over the last ten years? **Bill Madlock** of the Pittsburgh Pirates, of course, with close to a ten point lead over his nearest competitors, the unbelievable Pete Rose and Madlock's teammate Dave Parker. On the way he's won the NL batting crown four times (twice in Chicago), including the 1983 title and his 1975 .354 winner which is the highest one-season average in the Senior Circuit since 1971. Madlock loves to hit, and to eat —so much so that there is a weight clause in his contract and he's weighed once a month. "If I'm not 206 or under, I lose a substantial bonus. I'm five feet, eleven inches and my ideal weight is 205, so they haven't given me much of a margin. During the season I eat a very large breakfast, as I burn it off during the game. Unlike football, where they practice the whole week to prepare for the weekend game, in baseball we practice five percent of the time and play for the other ninety-five percent. When I get up (I usually sleep late), I'll have two glasses of freshly squeezed orange juice plus scrambled eggs mixed with cheese, six or seven slices of bacon and coffee. I don't eat again until after the game, and then it's usually another big meal. Steak, lobster, or veal and vegetables, preferably broccoli and corn."

Bill tries to avoid sugars and starches and never eats potatoes, but he will on occasion have fettucini as an appetizer if it's in the right restaurant. He also loves soufflés but generally sticks to fresh strawberries (his favorite fruit) and all kinds of melons. Sunday, however, is his day of sin. His wife makes him a special breakfast: four stacks of pancakes with maple syrup, three pancakes in each stack, eggs, bacon, fresh orange juice, and coffee. Off-season he cuts down at the table but continues to work out, playing tennis, racquetball, lifting weights, and exercising on a Nautilus machine. Breakfast is two glasses of fresh orange juice ("I must have it every day") with raisin bran and skim milk. A typical lunch is a small salad and soup, while dinner is simply steak or broiled chicken, and a steamed vegetable. Given his druthers, it could be a good deal more, but for Bill, the price is right.

**Willie Rändolph,** the Yankees All-Star second baseman, is both one of the fleetest and most nutritionally aware members of the team. He believes that a good diet will maximize his energy. In Randolph's case, this has not led him to any strange or unusual eating habits, just a serious consideration of which foods and in what amounts he should eat. Off-season and on travel days he doesn't normally have breakfast but he has a late brunch on the day of a game that consists of hominy grits with eggs and bacon. And while he may have been born in South Carolina, Randolph was raised from infancy in New York City, so his choice of grits is nutritional, not historical. At three o'clock before a night game he has a big dinner. This might consist of veal (his favorite is veal Parmesan) and noodles or spaghetti, with fruit for dessert. After the game he has a light supper of a sandwich with some ice cream. Randolph also takes a multi-vitamin each day, and if he still feels tired before a game he will have a spoonful of honey (which he keeps in his locker) for a quick energy boost to get him going until the adrenaline flow of playing takes over.

# In Training

The only time most fans see a Major League trainer in action is when he comes out with his little spray can of ethyl chloride to deaden the pain of one of his players who has just hit a screaming line drive off his instep. In fact, trainers' jobs are much more than just first aid. They are also the players' advisers on all physical therapies and training, including diet. **Jim Warfield,** the Cleveland Indians' trainer, is very high on the following one thousand and fifteen hundred calorie regimes, devised by the team's medical advisers, which are recommended according to the amount of weight loss or maintenance that is desired.

### ONE THOUSAND CALORIE DIET

Take one multi-vitamin each morning
fresh fruit, or canned—packed in own juice & drained
salads—use vinegar, lemon, or diet dressing

### Day One

| | |
|---|---|
| *Breakfast* | ½ cup unsweetened orange juice |
| | ¾ cup corn flakes |
| | ½ cup skim milk |
| *Snack* | small orange |
| *Lunch* | ½ cup cottage cheese |
| | 2 unsweetened peach halves |
| | carrot & celery sticks |

large glass ice tea—no sugar
4 graham crackers

*Snack*    1 cup tomato juice

*Dinner*    2 oz. broiled beef patty
1 cup plain carrots
salad—lettuce, tomato, cucumber
with vinegar
1 cup watermelon

*Snack*    1 cup skim milk

## Day Two

*Breakfast*    1 soft cooked egg
1 slice toast
1 tsp. jelly (no margarine)
½ grapefruit

*Snack*    small orange

*Lunch*    tuna salad   (½ cup drained tuna
(chopped celery & onion
(2 tsp. salad dressing
1 slice bread
dill pickles
ice tea—no sugar

*Snack*    2 graham crackers

*Dinner*    3 oz. plain baked chicken
½ cup mashed potatoes
½ cup plain green beans
salad—lettuce, tomato, cucumber
with vinegar

*Snack*    1 cup watermelon

70

## Day Three

*Breakfast*    ½ grapefruit
½ cup oatmeal
2 tbsps. raisins
½ cup skim milk

*Lunch*    egg salad  (1 egg, chopped
                        (chopped celery & onion
                        (2 tsp. salad dressing
1 slice bread
dill pickles
½ tomato
ice tea—no sugar

*Snack*

*Dinner*    3 oz. plain baked fish fillet
½ cup plain rice
½ cup plain broccoli
salad—lettuce, tomato, cucumber
with vinegar

*Snack*    1 cup skim milk
2 graham crackers

## Day Four

*Breakfast*    ½ cup grapefruit
1 slice toast, 1 tsp. jelly
(no margarine)
1 cup skim milk

*Lunch*    1 oz. cheddar cheese
6 saltine crackers
salad—½ tomato, ½ cucumber, lettuce
with vinegar
¾ cup strawberries
ice tea—no sugar

71

*Snack*        1 cup tomato juice
               3 thin three ring pretzels

*Dinner*       1 small to medium pork chop
               small baked potato, 1 tsp. margarine
               ½ cup plain sliced beets
               ½ tomato & onion salad
               with vinegar

*Snack*        1 cup milk (skim)
               2 graham crackers

## Day Five

*Breakfast*    ½ grapefruit
               1 soft cooked egg
               1 slice toast with 1 tsp. jelly

*Snack*        1 cup tomato juice

*Lunch*        2 oz. broiled beef patty
               salad—lettuce, cucumber, tomato
               with vinegar
               ½ cup pineapple

*Snack*        1 cup skim milk
               3 thin three ring pretzels

*Dinner*       3 oz. baked cod
               ½ cup mixed vegetables, plain
               salad as usual

*Snack*        ¼ cup cottage cheese with
               ½ cup pineapple

## Day Six

*Breakfast*    ½ cup orange juice
               1 scrambled egg cooked with 1 tsp.

72

margarine and 1 tsp. milk
1 slice toast with 1 tsp. jelly

*Lunch*          6 oz. vegetable soup
open face sandwich  (2 oz. lean ham
                    (1 slice tomato
                    (1 slice bread
¾ cup strawberries

*Snack*          1 cup tomato juice

*Dinner*         2 oz. meatballs, plain
½ cup spaghetti, 2 tbsp. tomato sauce
salad—tomato slices, cucumbers, lettuce
with vinegar
1 cup watermelon

*Snack*          ice tea—no sugar
small orange

## FIFTEEN HUNDRED CALORIE DIET

Take one multi-vitamin each morning
fresh fruit or canned—packed in own juice and drained
salads—use vinegar, lemon or diet dressing

### Day One

*Breakfast*      ½ medium grapefruit
soft boiled egg
1 slice bread
1 tsp. margarine
¾ cup plain dry cereal (corn flakes,
Cheerios, Wheaties, shredded wheat or
1 biscuit)
1 cup skim milk

*Lunch*          sandwich  (2 oz. lean roast beef
                    (2 tbsp. catsup
                    (2 slices bread
large glass ice tea, lemon

73

| | |
|---|---|
| *Dinner* | 4 oz. plain baked fish fillet<br>½ cup broccoli, 1 tsp. margarine<br>salad—tomatoes, cucumbers, lettuce<br>1 tbsp. salad dressing<br>1 slice bread, 1 tsp. margarine<br>2 peach halves |
| *Snack* | 1 cup skim milk<br>small orange |

## Day Two

| | |
|---|---|
| *Breakfast* | 1 cup unsweetened orange juice<br>2 slices toast<br>2 tsps. margarine<br>1 cup skim milk<br>coffee, tea—no sugar |
| *Lunch* | 6 oz. bowl vegetable soup<br>3 soda crackers<br>½ cup cottage cheese<br>⅓ cup canned fruit<br>ice tea, lemon, or diet soda |
| *Snack* | 1 cup skim milk<br>2 graham crackers |
| *Dinner* | 4 oz. baked chicken<br>1 cup plain carrots<br>1 small baked potato<br>1 tsp. margarine<br>salad—lettuce, cucumber, tomato<br>with vinegar |
| *Snack* | 1 cup low fat yogurt<br>(may substitute 1 cup milk for this)<br>2 peach halves |

## Day Three

Breakfast   ½ grapefruit
            1 cup oatmeal
            2 tbsps. raisins
            1 cup skim milk

Snack       1 banana

Lunch       2 oz. broiled beef patty (lean)
            1 hamburger bun
            dill pickles
            apple or orange

Dinner      spaghetti with meat sauce:
            (1 cup spaghetti with ¾ cup sauce
            2 tbsps. Parmesan cheese)
            salad—lettuce, cucumber, tomato
            ½ cup plain broccoli
            1 cup watermelon

Snack       1 cup skim milk
            4 graham crackers

## Day Four

Breakfast   ½ cup orange juice
            1 scrambled egg
            2 slices of toast (no butter or margarine)
            2 tsps. jelly or jam or honey
            1 cup skim milk

Snack       1 banana

Lunch       sandwich   (2 oz. low-fat cheese
                       (2 slices bread
                       (lettuce, tomato slice
                       (2 tsps. salad dressing
            orange or apple

*Snack*        1 cup skim milk

*Dinner*       3 oz. plain meat loaf
               ½ cup plain mashed potatoes
               1 cup plain spinach with vinegar if desired
               salad—lettuce, tomato, cucumber
               1 tbsp. salad dressing

*Snack*        apple

## Day Five

*Breakfast*    ½ grapefruit
               ¾ cup dry cereal
               ½ banana
               1 slice toast with jelly
               1 cup skim milk

*Lunch*        1 orange
               egg salad sandwich    (2 slices bread
                                     (1 egg chopped
                                     (chopped celery & onion
                                     (2 tsps. salad dressing
               dill pickles
               ice tea—no sugar

*Snack*        1 cup skim milk
               4 graham crackers

*Dinner*       4 oz. lean broiled steak
               1 cup green beans
               salad—lettuce, tomato, cucumber
               dinner roll—1 tsp. margarine
               1 cup tomato juice
               2 pear halves

76

## Day Six

Breakfast
½ cup unsweetened orange juice
½ cup oatmeal
2 tbsps. raisins
1 slice toast
1 tsp. margarine
1 cup skim milk

Lunch
1 hot dog
1 hot dog bun
mustard
¼ cup coleslaw
1 cup pineapple
dill pickles

Snack
1 cup skim milk
2 graham crackers

Dinner
4 oz. roast turkey
¼ cup sweet potato
½ cup mixed vegetables
salad—lettuce, tomato, cucumber
2 canned peach halves

## Day Seven

Breakfast
½ grapefruit
1 english muffin (or 2 slices toast)
2 tsps. margarine
1 poached egg
1 cup skim milk

Lunch
tuna fish sandwich (2 slices bread or 1 roll
(¼ cup drained tuna
(chopped celery & onion
(2 tsps. salad dressing
sliced tomato salad
dill pickles
1 cup skim milk

| | |
|---|---|
| *Snack* | apple or other fruit |
| *Dinner* | 3 oz. roast pork<br>1 small baked potato, 1 tsp. margarine<br>½ cup plain carrots<br>salad—lettuce, tomato, cucumber<br>1 banana |
| *Snack* | 4 graham crackers, hot tea |

## Day Eight

| | |
|---|---|
| *Breakfast* | ½ grapefruit<br>¾ cup dry cereal<br>2 tbsps. raisins<br>1 cup skim milk |
| *Lunch* | 1 cup broth<br>½ cup cottage cheese<br>2 peach halves<br>small lettuce salad<br>ice tea, plain |
| *Snack* | 1 cup skim milk<br>4 graham crackers |
| *Dinner* | 2 oz. baked ham<br>1 cup plain spinach with vinegar<br>½ cup plain rice<br>salad—as usual<br>1 cup pineapple |
| *Snack* | 1 cup yogurt, low fat, plain<br>½ cup fruit cocktail |

## Day Nine

| | |
|---|---|
| *Breakfast* | ½ cup orange juice<br>½ cup oatmeal, 2 tbsps. raisins |

|        |                                                                          |
|--------|--------------------------------------------------------------------------|
|        | 1 slice toast, 1 tsp. margarine<br>1 cup skim milk                       |
| *Lunch*  | ham sandwich  (2 slices bread<br>(2 oz. lean ham<br>(mustard, lettuce<br>½ cup yogurt, plain, low fat with<br>¼ cup regular fruit cocktail |
| *Snack*  | 1 orange<br>4 graham crackers                                            |
| *Dinner* | 3 oz. meat balls, plain<br>½ cup plain noodles<br>1 cup plain broccoli<br>salad as usual<br>1 cup watermelon |
| *Snack*  | 1 cup skim milk<br>1 oz. low fat American cheese<br>6 soda crackers      |

For those who don't want to follow a weekly plan, here are some basics (remember, though, the liquor and soft drink guidelines are limitations, *not* recommendations):

## CLEVELAND INDIANS REDUCTION DIET

Breakfast
    1 slice toast with butter or margarine
    1 egg
    1 glass milk
    Fruit—½ grapefruit *OR* one small glass orange juice *OR* one slice melon

Lunch
    1 sandwich (cold cuts, ham, hot dog)
    1 glass milk
    1 glass fruit juice *OR* 2 oranges *OR* 1 grapefruit

Dinner
> steak
> green salad
> 2 rolls (or bread)
> 1 glass milk
> ½ grapefruit

## REGULAR MEALS ARE IMPORTANT!!!

Additional Dietary Instructions

1) Eat any amount of these UNCOOKED vegetables that you wish.

| | | |
|---|---|---|
| asparagus | chicory | chard |
| broccoli | cucumber | collards |
| brussels sprouts | eggplant | dandelion |
| cabbage | escarole | kale |
| cauliflower | greens | mustard |
| celery | beet greens | poke |
| spinach | peppers | sauerkraut |
| turnip, greens | (green or red) | string beans, young |
| lettuce | radishes | squash, summer |
| mushrooms | romaine | tomatoes |
| okra | rhubarb | watercress |
| | (without sugar) | |

2) You may have two *DIET* soft drinks a day, *OR* if desired, two beers *OR* two cocktails.

3) You may have as much of the following as you desire:

| | | |
|---|---|---|
| coffee | lemon | mustard (dry) |
| tea | gelatin (unsweetened) | pickles (unsweetened) |
| clear broth | rennet tablets | saccharin and other |
| bouillon (fat free) | cranberries | noncaloric sweeteners |
| | (unsweetened) | |

pepper and other spices
vinegar
seasonings

It was historic Yankee domination that prompted the book and play about the Washington Senators' ("First in war, first in peace, last in the American League") revenge—*The Year the Yankees Lost the Pennant* or *Damn Yankees!* Well, they're making diet history now. George Steinbrenner decided early in the 1983 season to bring nutrition into the very heart of the ballpark, the clubhouse cafeteria. **Gene Monahan,** the Yankee trainer for the last eleven years, explains:

> We've gotten away from sugar and salt and all processed foods like cakes and candies. Sugar in the stomach can cause momentary muscular weakness. We also have gotten into the theory of glycogen reserves, what some people call carbohydrate loading, for our starting pitchers. That means eating a lot of pastas and pancakes and other easily digested carbohydrates two days before they are to play. For the other players, we no longer have donuts and danishes in the clubhouse for pregame snacks, rather things like raw uncooked vegetables, which add important roughage. We also have fruit to satisfy the sweet tooths, and dried fruit without sugar and unsweetened fruit juices instead of soda. We are not here to feed players, only to make their pregame nibbles more healthful. This is to give them some nutritious sustenance to carry into the game and some ideas about diet to follow on their own.

Here's the official snack menu (it is taken away two and one half hours before the game):

1. beverages
   canned unsweetened juices: apple, orange, peach nectar and apricot nectar
   2% low-fat milk
2. whole fruit: bananas, apples, oranges, plums, melon (cantaloupe or honeydew), pears
3. sherbet
4. freshly cut vegetables: celery, carrots, radishes, green peppers
5. whole wheat bread
6. assortments of fruit yogurt

7. all-natural dried fruit
8. on occasion, if there are extra long games: julienne salads made at the stadium with thin slices of ham and cheese and raw spinach instead of lettuce. Dressing is light vinegar.

If you were a Yankee and wanted advice from Monahan as to what to do to stay in shape off-season, he would hand you the following program (its use, of course, is not limited to the Bronx Bombers.):

*Off-Season Reducing Diet*

An off-season diet plan for the professional baseball player to lose weight and yet maintain certain metabolic and physical consistencies requires special considerations. This outline and model seven-day diet skeleton serves as a guide to you in whatever specific goals you have. Each man should discuss his goals and ideas with the team physician and trainer.

Crash dieting is out. Too many people have disrupted their normal body functions, lifestyles, and emotional states with the "crash diet" or so-called fad diets as the "water diet." Weight is lost yet so are vital nutrients needed for the body's organs to function efficiently. This outline will show that most normal foods are included and the most significant factors to be cognizant of are that here you will be eating two meals per day with *nothing* between meals, especially before bedtime. Also, it is the amount of caloric intake daily that will do the job for you. This is a gradual reduction diet that you can regulate yourself. Here you will be performing your normal daily routine (off-season), and managing on between two thousand and twenty-five hundred calories, as opposed to the three thousand plus recommended for seasonal play. The idea behind this plan is to eat sensibly and exercise, as you have scheduled your winter program.

There are three nutrients you consume. They are carbohydrates, protein, and fats. You need them *all* but as you will see, there will be a reduction in fatty food intake. Here again, this is a sensible plan for more often it is what "not to eat" that's the trick, as opposed to specifically what to eat. In addition to not eating between meals, beer is out and mixed drinks are to be taken at a minimum. These things, especially beer, are very high in calories and yet offer no food or bulk value. So be sensible here.

Following is an outline of a typical seven-day sensible plan. Substitute various items of the same type as you wish. Listed will be a "minor" meal plus a "major" meal for each of the seven days. Naturally, the major meal is to be eaten at the dinner hour in the late afternoon or evening, as opposed to the minor meal as a breakfast or lunch.

### Day One

*Minor meal*    4 oz. citrus juice (orange, grapefruit)
6 oz. serving whole grain cereal (milk or half-and-half)
1 slice toast (½ pat butter)
coffee, tea or 6 oz. 2% low-fat milk
1 whole fruit (orange, apple, banana, etc.)

*Major meal*    broth
light lettuce and tomato salad (low-calorie dressing)
8 oz. fat-trimmed shell steak or similar cut, broiled
1 medium baked potato (1 pat butter maximum)
6 oz. serving of green or white vegetable
4 oz. sherbet or Jell-O
no bread at this meal
coffee, tea, milk (6 oz. low-fat)

### Day Two

*Minor meal*    8–10 oz. bowl of soup (beef or vegetable stock)
1 sandwich (luncheon meat or spread)
lettuce, etc., permissible, but no butter

1 piece of fruit
8–10 oz. beverage (tea, milk, lemonade, etc.)

*Major meal*  fruit cup
portion of any size: fowl, chicken, turkey, etc.
boiled or baked potato (1 pat butter)
2 vegetables if desired (watch amount of salt and
butter added)
ice cream (6 oz.)
beverage as in minor meal

## Day Three

*Minor meal*  ¼ heart of lettuce salad (vinegar dressing or low-
cal commercial dressing)
beef or chicken chips on toast points
iced tea, coffee, low-fat milk
adult serving of gelatin dessert

*Major meal*  1 glass fruit juice
6 oz. broth soup
10 oz. serving of beef or calf's liver (no bacon)
6 oz. portion of white vegetable; cauliflower, corn,
potato
1 roll or slice of bread (½ pat butter)
beverage of choice

## Day Four

*Minor meal*  4 oz. fruit juice
two eggs scrambled
6 oz. ground chuck patty (broiled)
1 slice toast (1 pat butter)
8 oz. beverage of choice (2% low-fat milk, if
desired)

*Major Meal*  fruit cup
lettuce, tomato, onion salad
8–10 oz. portion of lean beef

green vegetable
3–5 oz. cottage cheese
mashed, baked, or broiled potato
sherbet, ice milk, or gelatin dessert
coffee, tea or 2% low-fat milk

## Day Five

*Minor meal*

protein plate consisting of
lettuce, boiled egg, sliced fish
carrot and celery sticks
cottage cheese
quartered tomato
beverage of choice
whole fruit

*Major Meal*

avocado salad
melon slice
fillet of fresh fish with lemon and margarine
6 oz. fresh vegetable
4 oz. ice cream with chocolate sauce

## Day Six

*Minor Meal*

unlimited citrus juice
6–8 oz. soup (beef, fowl, vegetable stock)
sandwich of choice (only two slices of bread)
sherbet (6 oz.) or piece of fruit
beverage of your choice

*Major Meal*

juice or fruit cup
cup of soup
breast of chicken, broiled or roasted
1 boiled potato (1 pat butter)
2 vegetables as desired
fruit cocktail

### Day Seven

*Minor meal*    6 oz. whole grain cereal with 2% low-fat
milk
1 English muffin or 2 slices toast (no more than 1
pat butter)
1 whole fruit
beverage of choice

*Major meal*    cottage cheese and celery and carrot sticks
braised short ribs of beef (10–14 oz. serving)
2 vegetables (6 oz. each)
2 dinner rolls or 1 slice of whole wheat bread (two
pats butter)
serving of fruit pudding, or ice cream
coffee, tea, diet soft drink, or 2% low-fat milk

Note that there is no real call for pastries or doughy desserts. Also, once or twice a week at most should you consume eggs. They are extremely high in cholesterol and have little place in your diet. Starchy foods of the Italian cuisine are not included although occasionally a meal of this type is not harmful if you use discretion.

*Hard* candy, a diet soft drink, or vegetable sticks may be taken moderately between meals. However, food of any type is to be avoided except for basics as mentioned. These mentioned will aid you in curbing your between meal appetite. At no time are medications to curb appetite to be employed. The team physician will answer all your questions along these lines. Also, fatty pork meats, such as bacon or sausage, have been totally eliminated. They serve you no real value in this diet concept.

This has been a rough sketch of a commonsense diet that will work for you if you obey the rules and exercise also. Just inquire as to substitutions you are in doubt about. This diet is very flexible. Remember that it's a two-meal-a-day program and to stay away from excessive, calorie-ridden foods.

*Sure Hits*

From famed sports eatery Oren & Aretsky in Manhattan, chef Steve Patino offers the following two recipes—definitely recommended to serve if Reggie Jackson or Ron Guidry are coming over for dinner.

An Oriental sauce accompanies grilled swordfish steaks in this spicy recipe favored by Reggie Jackson.

## GRILLED SWORDFISH STEAKS

Ingredients
2 swordfish steaks (7 oz.) rubbed with Oriental sesame oil
3 tbsps. of sesame oil
¼ cup of dry sherry
2 tbsps. of rice wine vinegar
4 tbsps. of soy sauce
¼ tsp. of sugar
1 pinch of cayenne pepper
2 tbsps. of thinly sliced scallions

Place the steaks on a very hot grill or Hibachi. After one or two minutes move them at a 90° angle on the same side to produce a crisscross grill mark.

The sauce may be cooked in a pan or used as a marinade one day before grilling. The ingredients are placed together and brought to a boil at which point a small knob of butter may be incorporated as a thickener.

The Yankees' ace, Cy Young Award winner Ron Guidry, is known as "Louisiana Lightning." Aside from Cajun cooking, this dish is at the top of his all-time list.

## SOFT SHELL CRABS MEUNIÈRE

Ingredients
4 medium (3 oz.) crabs, patted dry

3 tbsps. of fresh lemon juice
2 tbsps. of unsalted butter
1 tsp. of minced shallot
1 tbsp. of chopped parsley
¼ tsp. of freshly ground white pepper
1 pinch of salt

On a very hot skillet with clarified butter or oil, place the crabs underside down. Evenness of color is facilitated if they have been coated lightly with flour. When the crabs have become evenly browned, the oil must be drained from the pan which then may be placed in the oven at 450° for about five minutes, or until the crabs are crisp. To ensure crispness, the Meunière sauce should be made in the pan after the crabs have been removed.

The Meunière sauce is made by placing the above ingredients in order into the saucepan which should be very hot. Emulsification will then take place to produce a light and tangy sauce with a not too thick consistency.

# CHAPTER FOUR

# Football

Harsh physical contact has made football the only major team sport in America that remains an exclusively male domain, with no women's leagues or divisions at any significant level of play, fostering a particularly macho mystique. Nowhere is this more important than in the tough realities of line play, harking back to the unprotected head butting of the scrum in rugby. This is perhaps best illustrated by the probably apocryphal story of the ambulance ride shared by the gifted young wide receiver and the veteran defensive tackle following a tough game in the old AFL. As small talk, the rookie inquired as to his fellow traveler's reason for going to the hospital. He was regaled with a list of injuries to suit an entire orthopedic ward, topped by a broken thumb demonstrated by a bone protruding a quarter of an inch beyond the knuckle. When asked in return what brought him along, the youngster deftly changed the subject rather than admit to just a crushed rib.

Playing while hurt is still very much a part of the game, although reduced mobility is probably a bigger detriment than it used to be. Nevertheless, football, though a newer game, has changed much less than baseball over the last half century. It is still by and large a Saturday afternoon game in college and a Sunday one for the pros. The main difference now, however, is the platooning of offensive and defensive teams and the sophistication in passing offenses and defenses. By reducing playing time and providing better protective equipment, today's contact tends to score much higher on the Richter scale, in turn producing a new cottage industry around knee injuries. Of course, as with baseball, the other main change is economic. The only unions old-timers knew were the ones they joined to earn enough money off-season to afford playing professional football.

Also like today's baseball players, the modern star of the gridiron, although derided as a sissy by his predecessors for such affectations as face masks, are bigger, faster, and more mobile— and depend more on their diets to stay that way. Certainly, few would suggest that Lawrence Taylor deals out less punishing blows than any of the great linebackers of yesterday. Whether or not it's because he eats Captain Crunch for breakfast (except on game days) remains to be seen. Certainly Mark Gastineau attributes his strength and quarterback sacking quickness in part to the special protein drink he's concocted.

Here are some of the other diet tips, secrets, and recipes of great ballplayers past and present plus advice from medical men and trainers for the New York Giants, Dallas Cowboys, and Washington Redskins.

# In the Trenches:
# The Linemen

The Cincinnati Bengals' All-Pro offensive tackle **Anthony Munoz** at six feet, six inches and 270 pounds is one of the great physical specimens in the National Football League. While one sports professional spoke of him in awe as a "building," I prefer to think of him as something nice in a three bedroom townhouse. To defensive linemen he just means trouble, and he's equally as resolute a blocker of food he considers unhealthy. "God gave me the natural ability to play," he says, "but I've helped it along by being aware of nutrition. I started learning about it in college and after that it was just a matter of applying it." He uses no salt and avoids using butter. In addition, Munoz and his wife are label readers. "We read everything before we buy it and stay away from any preservatives, sodium, and sugar. The only fattening thing we eat is ice cream, but that's only on occasion. Most of the things I eat are either baked or broiled. If I have cold cereal it will be something like Shredded Wheat, not the sugared kind. Fruit juices come from the health food store and my favorites are lemon lime, mandarin lime, or grapefruit made by Hansons. They are carbonated and made with fructose instead of white sugar and taste like soda. I run a minimum of four miles a day but the last couple of years it's usually been six miles. If I get cramps, I'll eat bananas for potassium. Gatorade makes me thirstier, so I'll just have water with ice."

For breakfast, Munoz has a bowl of mixed fruit consisting of grapefruit, oranges, and apples along with a cup of coffee. He doesn't like eating before a game, preferring to play on an empty stomach. After the game, however, he will go out with his teammates and have a salad, steak, and potatoes, or chicken and rice, and an occasional glass of wine.

The secret to dieting, he feels, is to change your eating habits. "Shortcuts like powder diets and quick weight loss plans work for a limited amount of time and then you just put everything back on again. You must go out and run, get plenty of exercise and eat in moderation, and also make a chart of everything you put in your mouth to see what you're doing wrong." And as far as defensive linemen are concerned, in Munoz's case, it's not much.

At left anchor of the New York Sack Exchange, the Jets' **Mark Gastineau** is best known throughout the league for his celebratory dances following each of his numerous sacks. What keeps him light on his feet is a diet that does not include bread. "I've found by trial and error that a high protein diet works for me," he said, "and I stay away from all refined sugars and starches." His diet throughout the day both during and off-season is dominated by eggs, fish, chicken, and red meat. "When I was younger I was overweight," he recalls, "and I learned over the years by watching others. It's amazing how little people understand about nutrition. That's probably why they don't feel guilty about what they're eating."

Gastineau says he's in better shape off-season because of a strict program of weight-lifting, racquetball, and basketball. "I find that protein builds up the muscles that the weights tear down." He also takes liquid protein in his favorite flavor, black cherry, and if he's very tired he'll whip up a special high-energy drink. The recipe is quite simple: put two glasses of freshly squeezed orange juice into a blender and add two tablespoons of protein powder and ice cubes. It's a concoction sure to get you out of the sack, even if not guaranteed to produce them.

The offensive captain and right tackle of the Giants, Stanford educated **Gordon King** is a thinking man's lineman. His diet is equally thoughtful. "Nutrition is extremely important in the life of an athlete," he feels. "It is a highly neglected area and sooner or later eating junk food will catch up to you. The most important thing is to stay as natural as possible, although today it is getting to be a challenge to find high quality food. I get a lot of help from my wife Susan, who is a vegetarian and very conscious of using fresh ingredients."

King also prefers to play on an empty stomach. Therefore, four hours before the game he eats just a baked potato and some fruit—oranges, apples, bananas, or melon. Fruit, he feels, is easily digestible and a good source of carbohydrates. The rest of his preparations are equally planned. "If you're tired on a game day," he says, "you're in a lot of trouble. Sundays, the body is pumped full of adrenaline. The most important night's sleep is on Friday before a Sunday game, and then I try to get at least eight hours." Saturdays are spent relaxing as much as possible. After the game, however, he might have a steak or chicken or his usual dinner staple, fish, plus a beer to relax. The rest of his post-game meal is pretty standard fare for him—a large fresh salad, vegetables, a baked potato or brown rice, and more fruit for dessert. During the week, King's diet is less traditional. "I don't believe in cholesterol. Junk foods have a higher count of it than eggs, for example." Three or four times a week his breakfast will be hard boiled eggs plus a slice of whole wheat toast (he never eats processed white bread, always the whole grain type) with sunflower margarine, never butter. One dish that he likes is based on protein rich tofu. "Put a colander on top of a cake of tofu and drain the water out. Then cut it into strips and stir-fry it in some safflower oil until golden brown. Add ginger, garlic, and some strips of steak and you have a wonderful high protein dinner." For vitamins, King takes a multiple time-release with minerals, a B complex plus extra $B_1$, $B_6$, and $B_{12}$, forty grains of brewer's yeast, sixty to one hundred grains of desiccated liver plus lecithin. He also likes supplements such as papaya, acidophilus, and alfalfa, and if he gets a sprain, he'll take comfrey root to alleviate it.

King is confident his regime works for him. When he starts training camp again he can really feel it: "It's like boot camp with contracts," he says. "It's a grind. But due to eating well I feel fresher than the others." Tofu, comfrey tea, and safflower oil—not too long ago pro football players wouldn't even have heard of these, not to mention eat them. But then again, at six feet, six inches and 275 pounds, no one is going to make fun of King's choice of comestibles.

Other than the Dallas Cowboys, the only people happy to see **Ed "Too Tall" Jones** back in uniform at defensive end were the boxers he would have fought if he had continued his alternate professional sporting career of pugilism. At six feet, nine inches and 265 pounds, Jones might be too tall but he clearly isn't too heavy. To keep in such good proportion he has definite ideas about good nutrition. "I eat very little food generally and at game time I prefer to have nothing in my stomach. When it's hot out, I'll just have a glass of carrot juice before the game." In the colder weather, he eats something a little more substantial, like an egg or a small strip of steak.

Like Gastineau, Jones believes in a high protein diet to maintain his energy, rather than carbohydrates. His lunches generally consist of tuna salad with sliced tomatoes, while dinners are broiled chicken or fish, but little red meat. He will have this with a few vegetables, his favorites being carrots and spinach, and a small salad. Jones eats no sweets at all and will not even have too much fruit because of its high sugar content. He also does not eat bread, only crackers, but occasionally during the season he'll have some spaghetti for extra carbohydrates. His favorite meal of all, though, is little bitty chicken wings.

**Joe Greene** is no longer Mean now that he's retired from his years as the main support of Pittsburgh's vaulted Steel Curtain. The preeminent defensive tackle of his day, Greene has four Super Bowl rings to show for it. While his games against the Cowboys were classics, he remains true to his Texas roots when it comes to cuisine. In fact, his restaurant, The Dallas Partners, specializes in Texican food, and Greene's favorite dinner in the world is a combination called Muy Loco. This consists of a plate of nachos, chili, cheese, refried beans, guacamole, and sour cream topped off with jalapeño peppers and washed down with a mug of beer. Maybe that's what made him mean to start with.

At six feet, four inches, Greene doesn't really have to worry about his weight. Nevertheless, he eats only one meal a day. "I love to eat, but if I eat three meals one day, the next day I will fast. I try to count calories and I know what my body reacts to. I tried all kinds of diets but I have developed a certain discipline over the years and one meal a day works perfectly. I also don't take vitamins as I found that they increased my appetite. I don't really exercise anymore; I did for twenty years and now I'm all burnt out on exercise." Fortunately he has also given up cheesecake, pecan pie, and beer, "but my weakness is Bluebell's Cookies and Cream ice cream. The foods I eat for feeling well and fit are chicken, veal, lobster, lamb—and all types of seafood. If I eat chicken, I take all the skin off. The vegetables I like are cabbage, spinach, and asparagus. A steak, salad, and a glass of wine are also a great dinner for me. My ideal breakfast is waffles made with eggs, flour, and butter."

Greene is another superstar who was in the forefront of discovering the benefits of building up glycogen reserves. "I guess the secret for young players is eating more carbohydrates. When I was playing I would load up on them, the breads and pastas. It's also a good tip for traveling. Twenty-four to forty-eight hours before a game carbohydrates allow you to go in strong but feel light—even traveling over two time zones. They get burned up quicker." Greene also believes in letting a well-tuned body rule the diet. "Actually, the secret is to have fun, to enjoy what you're eating. It's funny in football, the guys who were trying to be big ate health food, and the big ones were able to eat anything they wanted."

# Heavy Armor:
# The Linebackers

Voted the NFL's top defensive player in both 1981 and 1982 and one of the few defenders who have forced opponents into adjusting their game plan around him, the New York Giants' All-Everything outside right linebacker **Lawrence Taylor** has to be considered the best at his position in football. The word "awesome" comes most readily to mind. At six feet, two inches and 237 pounds, Taylor may like to experiment with his pass rushing technique but not with his food. "I stick to certain basic things, and though I'm not a health nut, I don't eat sugar and have a set diet that I know will make me feel and play well." For example, the only kinds of fruit he'll eat are apples and oranges. In fact, if he's tired he'll just eat an orange for quick energy. If he's very tired, he'll take a nap—although there are a whole bunch of opposing players who will swear that either pro ball doesn't tire him or he takes some pretty ferocious naps in the fourth quarter. Taylor is another player who doesn't eat white bread, only raisin pumpernickel, whole wheat and corn bread. He avoids seafood and bananas, though not out of nutritional concerns, but because he had to eat them as a kid and *no one* is going to make him now.

The night before a game he'll have a steak, potatoes, and lots of dark leafy vegetables like collard greens. Taylor believes that in his case beer helps him to perspire and feel loose, so he'll also have a few beers that evening. His theory is that the combination of protein, carbohydrates, and vitamins and minerals will digest overnight and be available for use the next afternoon at game time. The next morning he'll have only a large glass of orange juice. He always plays on an empty stomach.

On nongame days, Taylor has a large breakfast consisting of cereal, eggs, bacon, and toast. If he gets up late he eats just cereal for lunch. Off-season when he travels he tends to eat more because of luncheons and dinner events, and he usually puts on more weight. He doesn't like jogging to stay in shape, but does play basketball. Presumably, few court opponents try to fight through one of his picks—at least not twice. When the season starts again, he brings his own fruit to training camp and drinks lots of liquids, mainly water and milk. "When I was younger I had a weight problem. So over the last few years, I have become much more careful about what I eat."

The Dallas Cowboys' man in the middle is **Bob Breunig,** voted the NFC's top middle linebacker after the 1980 season. He is a firm believer in keeping fit. A Pro Bowler, Breunig builds for the gridiron by exercising during the off-season. He jogs two miles five days a week, lifts weights three days and runs wind sprints two days. He also plays racquetball and basketball, swims, and water skis. It is easy to pick out Breunig at training camp—he's the one who isn't perspiring.

The law at the Breunigs' is no junk food, soda pop, packaged food, or sweetened desserts during the week. Breunig adds: "I also limit fat intake, watch sugar, white flours, packaged and preserved foods, prepared cakes, and caffeine. In fact, I feel better not eating any sugar at all. I also stay away from fried foods and heavy butter sauces. On the plus side, I eat steamed vegetables, and balance this with proper protein, although I limit my red meat. In order to get enough protein I do eat meat and drink milk since I found I need protein for strength. This is okay if it's balanced with vegetables and fruit and carbohydrates. Too many people just eat steak and eggs."

For breakfast Breunig has one or two slices of whole grain toast and a bowl of whole grain cereal—granola, Raisin Bran or Shredded Wheat. Or, he has one or two eggs, fruit, and fruit juice. Lunch is a large sandwich, usually turkey, on whole grain bread, with lettuce and tomatoes (for roughage), fresh cheese (calcium), and a yogurt. In between, he drinks a lot of water and snacks on apple, grapefruit, or orange juice. Dinner is a meat dish with fresh vegetables and a large salad with all kinds of fresh vegetables mixed in. "I love broccoli, spinach, carrots, cucumbers, tomatoes, and potatoes, although I have a little trouble with okra. Thursday through Sunday I have my own special regime, call it superstition if you want, but it's always worked. Thursday and Friday nights I'll have a good sized steak, baked potato, and a salad. On Saturday, when I wake up I'll have a doughnut and milk for breakfast and a big hamburger for lunch. Dinner is spaghetti with tomato sauce and garlic bread. Before bed I'll have a root beer float, sixteen ounces of root beer and vanilla ice cream. The next morning I will have French toast (dipped in egg) and a large glass of fresh juice. The key word is discipline. I find I burn off this carbohydrate packing during the game and I keep pretty fit throughout the week."

**Brad Van Pelt** is one of those rare athletes who was seriously courted by two major sports. The former Wolverine pitcher became a New York Giant, though, when that meant only football. This All-Pro linebacker's sporting interests are not limited to just baseball and football, however. He is also the owner of a golf club in his home state of Michigan called, appropriately, Club 10.

His diet is equally well-rounded. At six feet, five inches and 235 pounds, down from 250, Van Pelt relies on quickness and has to watch his weight. As a result, he eats a lot of fish and chicken and tries to stay away from red meat. On a game day he'll eat no breakfast at all, since, like his confrere Taylor, he likes to play with an empty stomach. Right after the game he has shrimp, lobster, or any kind of broiled fish or chicken. Van Pelt used to eat fish and fowl fried instead of broiled, but he has learned that broiling makes for lighter and more easily digestible meals. He will only occasionally eat steak or roast beef. The team wants him to play at 235 and he has found it harder to keep slim on a red meat diet. And as far as alcohol is concerned, Van Pelt seems to have all the options covered except perhaps for dropping three potential interceptions in a Giants' win: "The only time I drink is for celebrations or drowning my miseries after the game, then I will have beer or a screwdriver."

In the off-season, Van Pelt plays a lot of golf and eats more red meat. Lunch will be at the clubhouse of Club 10 and then it will be chicken salad or tunafish sandwiches. His favorite meals include the ones cooked by his mother—especially breaded ham made by frying ham dipped in a batter made from eggs and crackers. Some allegiances are more important than team and diet.


# Assault Troops:
# Receivers and Backs

Generally considered to be the most reliable wide receiver in the game right now, **Dwight Clark's** most memorable catch was probably the one that won the NFC Championship game against Dallas, which enabled San Francisco to go on to win Super Bowl XVI, capping a brilliant season for the 49ers. Joe Montana's favorite target, Clark has an almost uncanny ability to find the weakness in a defense. The only weakness in his diet, however, is the banana and mayonnaise sandwiches on white bread that were made by his Aunt Bee when he was growing up in Georgia. He also has a strong liking for peanut butter and banana sandwiches.

Clark, however, has recently changed his ideas on nutrition with the help of Jerry Attaway, the team's nutritionist. "Before, I felt that you needed a big steak before a game to give you energy. But then a lot of times during a game I started to get dizzy. I realized that I had nothing to stay with to keep going." Now he prepares for the game by starting two days before: He'll eat potatoes, rice, or pasta—his favorite being cheese melted on noodles. "Carbohydrates are what you burn," he says, "and they make you move faster and feel lighter." The Friday before the game he'll practice all day and he'll bring his own sandwich to the practice. This will consist of tuna or turkey on whole grain bread. Saturday night before the game he'll load up on pasta, another favorite being fettucini Alfredo, plus whole grain bread. On the morning of the game he'll have half a pancake and half a piece of toast. After the game, usually about five or six o'clock, he'll have fish or chicken, or occasionally red meat, plenty of fresh vegetables, and "lots of beer." He never drinks coffee and only drinks

skim milk, which has less fat than whole but more carbohydrates per ounce, and quarts of orange juice.

Off-season Clark plays golf and tennis and, presumably for
the purpose of increasing his vitamin D content, lies out in the
sun. Three times a week he lifts weights and runs sprints. This
new program has given him more strength and stamina. "I used
to have to chew dextrose tablets during a game to keep going.
Now nothing stops me."

One of football's all-time greatest running backs, **Walter
Payton** has almost single-handedly kept the Monsters of the
Midway fearsome. A slashing runner with blazing speed, Payton has moves that keep the memory of Gale Sayers alive in
Chicagoan hearts. There is only one thing alive whose claws
Payton cannot escape. No, it is not the *Linebackerus ferocious.* It
is instead the *Homarus americanus.* Lobster is his favorite food
—prepared almost any way. He'll have it for dinner whenever
he can.

Payton's other meals are much more suited to a speedster
than the slow moving denizen of the deep he favors. Breakfast
is balanced and solid (as is five foot, ten inch, 202 lb. Payton),
either eggs and bacon, French toast, or pancakes with orange or
pineapple juice. Lunch is light, usually a large salad. Like his
running style, Payton's diet has no weaknesses.

Heisman Trophy winner **Herschel Walker** is the big gun of
the USFL's New Jersey Generals, who look for him to do for
their league what famed nutritionist Broadway Joe Namath did
for the AFL. While only a youngster by football standards, his
diet echoes that of the veterans.

Walker has no trouble at all maintaining his six-foot, six-
inch, 220-pound frame. "The only time I eat is at dinner around
seven o'clock and then it will be a steak, a hamburger, or some
chicken. If I have anything else it will be some soup, like French
onion, and occasionally a baked potato. The only fruit I eat is
oranges. I don't have a pregame meal or even breakfast on the
morning before a game. I don't like the feeling of having anything in my stomach. Candy and cookies are my weakness but
I feel I burn them up." But basically Walker's diet results from
his lack of interest in eating, rather than nutritional concerns.

"I don't think about food at all," he says. "My energy is God-given. It doesn't come from what I eat."

# The Air Force:
# QBs and Kickers

Handing off to Franco Harris or Rocky Bleier and passing to the likes of Lynn Swan and John Stallworth may make a quarter-back's life a whole lot easier, but leading your team to four Super Bowls isn't done with mirrors. **Terry Bradshaw,** the only QB who has managed the feat, also knows the need to stay light on his feet. "I don't eat one bit of food after five o'clock on Saturday night, although Sunday night after the game I eat the biggest pizza I can find. I pass a pizza parlor on my way home after the game and I can't resist ordering their larg-est pepperoni. I feel I can afford (and need) this binge since I tend to lose eight or nine pounds each game in any case. However, during the week it's all fish and chicken, either baked, broiled or barbecued, along with mashed potatoes and green beans. I also adore onions and will eat them any way possible." A new secret weapon against onrushing line-men?

Bradshaw's other favorite vegetables include asparagus, cab-bage, tomatoes, and corn. "I also love a vegetable goulash I make with corn, peas, onions, garlic, and a touch of sugar. I mix this all together and have it with corn bread and chicken on the side and it's my idea of heaven. My ideal way to start out the day is to have an enormous breakfast consisting of six eggs, two glasses of milk, six pieces of toast, and about a pound of bacon, and then not eat anything else until the next day. Unfortunately, my schedule is such that I have to leave for practice early in the morning and I really don't have enough time to eat anything, so I settle for dinner at six o'clock. The reason I prefer to eat a big breakfast is that you burn it all off during the day and I sleep much better on a totally empty stomach." Bradshaw's lack of sleep must be contagious. Over the years he's given plenty of defenders nightmares.

As the brilliant young quarterback of the Minnesota Vikings, **Tommy Kramer** has done the impossible—made Viking fans, if not forget, at least not miss Fran Tarkenton. One of the flashiest passers in the game, Kramer keeps his lanky six foot, two inch, 205 pound body in shape by eating lightly. For breakfast he has a glass of orange juice followed by cold cereal and a glass of milk, while lunch is simply a tuna, ham, or egg salad sandwich. Dinner is a bit more substantial, with some solid protein, usually a steak, salad, and plenty of fresh vegetables, his favorites being broccoli, carrots, string beans, asparagus, and peas. He loves barbecue and will either grill a small steak or experiment with different types of chicken dishes. His pregame meal on Saturday night always consists of steak, green beans, a baked potato, and fruit salad. And even with this balanced diet, he takes vitamins E, A, and B complex along with extra calcium and liquid lecithin daily.

Another ice cream lover, Kramer doesn't eat it often. "When I was younger I had a hard time putting on weight, but now I have to watch it or I'll gain." Off-season his diet remains about the same, and to keep up with the calories he has a strict exercise regime: lifting different weights for three days, throwing for four days, and running for one and a half miles every day. Dodging defensive linemen is a year-round effort.

Not only the quarterback of America's Team, **Danny White** is the only pro quarterback who plays a dual role, being also the Cowboys' punter. No other pro is called on to regularly exercise both hand-to-eye and foot-to-eye coordination or is as proficient at both. Always among the top rated passers, White has thrived under pressure both for replacing Roger Staubach and working on the combination pressure cooker and glass bowl that is the Dallas Cowboys. White feels that the body thrives on good nutrition. "You might get away with eating junk food while you're young," he says "but you'll feel it eventually."

For breakfast, White has a bowl of whole grain wheat cereal that is imported from Canada. He boils the whole grains in water, and has the hot mixture with a piece of whole wheat toast. Or he'll eat an omelette. For extra vitamins, White takes a handful every day that are put together in a Sports Pac by Neo Life. Lunch (other than on game days—he won't eat within four hours of game time) is eaten on the run and it's usually a barbecue plate of beef with vegetables and cole slaw. For dinner he likes chicken or hamburgers and sometimes has the chicken in a variety of casseroles. He'll always have plenty of fresh vegetables, his favorites being squash, broccoli, corn, and peas. Brown rice and salad with Thousand Island dressing might round out the meal, when his willpower remains strong. His weakness is desserts, however, and whenever he can get away with it he'll have a hot-fudge sundae with chocolate-chip cookies. But that's not often; usually he's extremely careful and won't eat any dessert at all.

**Dave Jennings,** football's premier punter, modestly minimized his contributions by claiming that all he does is run on the field, kick, and run off. But the value of booming one out amid a maze of onrushing would-be blockers over and over again to pin the other team deep in its territory is not underestimated by any Giant fan. Jennings is the important twelfth man to their imposing defense.

At six feet, five inches and 190 pounds, Jennings is also careful to maintain the litheness that gives his leg kick its great velocity. To that end he is a light eater. He has a very large glass of orange juice in the morning and then doesn't eat again until late in the day. From nine-thirty to four-thirty he works out: three times a week he lifts weights and every day does some kind of cardiovascular work such as running, basketball, riding either a stationary or a fourteen-speed bike, or racquetball. Afterward for dinner, he will eat chicken or red meat (he loves prime ribs), and a salad, but no potatoes or vegetables and bread only once in a while. He does love fruit, however, and will have all kinds of melon, especially cantaloupe, honeydew, and watermelon. It is only on game day that he breaks this rhythm—four hours before a game he will have French toast with maple syrup. To balance his diet, Jennings takes a multiple vitamin supplement both in the morning and in the evening plus lots of vitamin C, five thousand milligrams a day.

# Corps Men

**Dr. Alan Levy,** team doctor for the New York Giants (and the New Jersey Nets), is obviously a leading authority on athletes and their diets. He has been campaigning to increase their nutritional awareness and habits, with mixed success.

> It's been a fight to try to change the pregame meal. Athletes are basically very superstitious, if something works for them they don't want to change it. The younger ones, however, are much more aware of good nutrition. Before, the players only wanted a steak and a salad, but no butter or milk. Steak is not good because it is low in carbohydrates. It is fine to eat after the game, but before, the high fat content slows the emptying time. It is better to have something such as pancakes and syrup or waffles and syrup. Simple carbohydrates work the best with a moderation of sugar. During a game the players can burn up to seven thousand calories so they better have something in them to burn. If you eat well you do not need to load up on vitamins. In fact, one multiple a day is enough for most people. When I started everyone wanted $B_{12}$ shots, then vitamin E, now they want $B_{15}$ which is supposed to increase endurance. Your body can build a tolerance to vitamin C as well. My theory is to eat a good balanced diet, staying away from alcohol and caffeine. There's only one problem, the superstitious ones who feel that if it has worked well for them before, it's a ritual and they will not deviate. If I introduce something new to them, I hope it works because after that they will stick to it.

**Bob Ward,** the conditioning coach for the Dallas Cowboys, has a simple philosophy. Its five elements are: "Dream great dreams. Find out where you are in relation to these dreams. Construct a game plan to reach your dreams. Start now. Never quit." All this can be applied to his nutritional philosophy along with one additional rule: "The three things to remember for a healthy life are work, rest, and nutrition. All of these have to be in proper sync, however. For example, if the work load is increased, so must the nutrition and the rest. If decreased, less food is needed and less rest as well. Everything must be in proportion. Athletes just work more; that's how they differ from the layman. As far as nutrition is concerned, it must be a cross-section of foods with nutritional benefits. We should reach a point where our bodies will tell us what the rules are. The choice is ours, but our body will tell us if we just listen." And it is not limited to football players. When I interviewed Arnold Schwarzenegger a few years back he had a similar philosophy, "If you take care of your body, it will tell you if it has any special needs—once it's in tune. If you have a sudden craving for sugar, for example, have some and don't worry about it. It just means that your body needs it at the moment. A healthy body takes care of itself." Ward agrees. We must reeducate ourselves, he feels. "A powerful predictor for success is commitment. Those who are committed to health habits are the ones that will find the answers. If anything detracts from your performance, you will not be living up to your potential. Performance equals potential minus any losses due to faulty process. If there is anything negative, you will be performing at a sub-maximum level. If you eat junk food, you are introducing negatives to your body and will not be performing well." Ward really sounds like a coach. If any of his players don't get his message, you know it can only be because he just wasn't listening.

**Bubba Tyre** had the rare pleasure of being the trainer for a Super Bowl winning team, XVII's Washington Redskins. While he does not claim all the credit, Tyre does feel that nutrition plays an important role in performance. "My responsibility as a trainer is to keep the players in good shape. They are fined if they don't record their weights every day. I always recommend that the players eat a great breakfast and work it off. Most players can lose up to twelve pounds of fluid just in a practice. On the training table we set out pancakes, waffles, toast, potatoes, fresh fruit, and fresh fruit juices, but no milk as it can cause an upset stomach. Lunch is fresh soup, cold cuts, turkey, chicken, roast beef, watermelon, more fruit juices, and a salad bar. Dinner is the main protein meal, and now the trend is to eat less red meat, and more chicken and fish."

For getting ready for games during the season, Tyre is another devotee of carbohydrates: "The body can use up carbohydrates faster. Therefore, now in the pregame meals we stress eating four hours before playing and we now tell players the importance of things like French toast and waffles. Vitamins are not really important if they eat the proper foods. A good breakfast is always important. A good tip for young players is to avoid sodas, try instead taking two thirds water and one third Gatorade poured over fresh orange or grapefruit juice. This restores both the lost fluids and electrolytes and is a real pick-me-up as well." On a team famed for Hogs and Smurfs, it's good to know that their diet at least is human.

**Ronnie Barnes,** trainer of the Giants, is a serious student of his players and their needs. "We encourage the players to eat protein, carbohydrates, and some fats, and drink plenty of water. At training camp we can closely watch the players and can monitor what they are eating and what they should be eating. I am most concerned about the fat intake of some players. The ones that eat hamburgers and ice cream, for example, are ingesting too much fat. We try to teach them about food substituting—pancakes, spaghetti, and French toast can be substituted for hamburgers and steaks, for example. I also recommend baked potatoes, another food that is nutritious and supplies carbohydrates, which translates into energy. Honey is also outstanding and we always keep it available to the players. During warm weather I stress bananas, which are high in potassium, along with other fruit such as apples, grapes, and plums."

Despite his linebackers' preferences, Barnes espouses what seems to be the majority view: "We find it is good to eat about four hours before a competition. Players psychologically feel better if they can put something in their mouths and then chew on it. Besides, liquid diets can give diarrhea. It is okay to supplement with them, but not for a meal in itself.

"Another important point to remember in any pregame plan is to stick to things that you are familiar with. One player I knew had a two o'clock Italian banquet the day before a game with clams casino, mussels, etc., and had an incredible gastrointestinal upset at game time. Some players have a lactose intolerance. They have to watch out for things like rice pudding, which is a popular dessert that they may not immediately associate with milk. In general, I recommend that the players stay away from greasy food, which is hard to digest. Anything heavy or intolerable combines instantly with the excitement and nerves of the game." For those who wake up ill, Barnes's advice is that warm tea helps as does ginger ale. "I also recommend a clear fluid diet for someone with stomach problems on the day of a game; eat only foods you can see through, bouillon, water, Jell-O, ginger ale—even chicken soup. Also the more energy you expend, the more you'll have to take in to maintain your energy. The best source of vitamins is from your diet."

There is nothing transparent, however, about the strong bias toward carbohydrates and protein in the training table diet planned for the Giants by **Dick Rossi,** Assistant Director of Operations of the Food Service Department at the University of Massachusetts. Remember though that this regime is designed for *extremely* active and very large young men who have to be psychologically pleased as well. Many of the dishes included are not on Barnes's list of recommended foods, but are served to accommodate the long-standing habits of many of the players. As Merle Best, the Giants' nutritionist points out, change in diet is extremely hard to introduce to men engaged in a very stressful situation. Along with Barnes, she is trying to slowly win them over to modern nutritional theories, especially weaning them from excessive animal protein, fat and fried foods in favor of complex carbohydrates, but they do not want to unnecessarily annoy any 270-pound tackles in the process.

## THE NEW YORK GIANTS' TRAINING TABLE

### Sunday

*Breakfast*        scrambled eggs
pancakes
fried eggs
sausage

| | |
|---|---|
| *Lunch* | grilled ham/cheese<br>shrimp creole<br>french fries |
| *Dinner* | baked ham<br>spaghetti w/meat balls—garlic bread<br>green beans<br>peas and carrots<br>sweet potatoes |

## Monday

| | |
|---|---|
| *Breakfast* | scrambled eggs<br>poached eggs<br>French toast<br>bacon<br>pastry |
| *Lunch* | beef noodle soup<br>California quiche<br>club sandwich |
| *Dinner* | prime ribs<br>Cornish game hen with rice stuffing<br>chopped kale<br>buttered corn<br>baked potato with sour cream |

## Tuesday

| | |
|---|---|
| *Breakfast* | scrambled eggs<br>fried eggs<br>pancakes<br>sausage |
| *Lunch* | tomato soup<br>shepherd's pie<br>Italian sausage wedge with peppers & onions<br>wax and green beans |

| | |
|---|---|
| *Dinner* | roast leg of lamb with mint jelly |
| | manicotti with French bread |
| | home-fried potatoes |
| | tiny whole carrots |
| | chopped broccoli |

## Wednesday

| | |
|---|---|
| *Breakfast* | scrambled eggs |
| | cheese omelette |
| | French waffles |
| | grilled ham slices |
| | |
| *Lunch* | chicken noodle soup |
| | broccoli/cauliflower casserole |
| | Philadelphia steak sandwich |
| | lima beans |
| | |
| *Dinner* | bread fried chicken quarter |
| | meatloaf with gravy |
| | baked fillet of sole |
| | rice pilaf |
| | green beans bretonne |
| | stewed tomatoes |

## Thursday

| | |
|---|---|
| *Breakfast* | scrambled eggs |
| | boiled eggs—hard/soft |
| | fritters with syrup |
| | bacon |
| | |
| *Lunch* | vegetable soup |
| | baked macaroni and cheese |
| | bacon, lettuce & tomato wedge |
| | carrots in orange sauce |
| | |
| *Dinner* | 16 oz. broiled strip steak with mushroom sauce |
| | eggplant Parmesan |

baked potato with sour cream
fresh broccoli
mixed vegetables

## Friday

*Breakfast*   scrambled eggs
fried eggs
French toast
sausage patty

*Lunch*   vegetable beef soup
hot turkey sandwich with gravy
baked ziti
creamed corn

*Dinner*   steamship round
baked haddock with Newburg sauce
parslied boiled potatoes
buttered peas
Harvard beets

## Saturday

*Breakfast*   scrambled eggs
mushroom omelette
blueberry pancakes
ham

*Lunch*   chicken rice soup
hamburger on sesame-seed bun
cheeseburger
liver and onions
French fries
buttered peas

*Dinner*   shish kebob
fisherman's platter (fried fish, fried clams, fried shrimp, cole slaw, fries)

    leaf spinach
    sliced yellow squash
    tiny whole potatoes

# Kitchen Maneuvers

Bob Breunig's wife, Mary, has organized a cookbook of the Dallas Cowboys' favorite recipes. Here are some samples:

"TD" **Tony Dorsett** has blazed through the record books and astonished would-be tacklers both at the University of Pittsburgh and Dallas with magic moves. This dish is about the only thing guaranteed to keep him in one place.

### TONY DORSETT'S SOUR CREAM MARINATED CHICKEN BREASTS

    1 carton sour cream (8 oz.)
    ¼ cup lemon juice
    2 tsps. Worcestershire sauce
    2 tsps. celery salt
    1 tsp. paprika
    2 cloves garlic, minced
    2 tsps. pepper
    5 whole chicken breasts, split
    salt
    bread crumbs
    ½ cup butter or margarine, melted
    ¼ cup shortening, melted

Combine sour cream, lemon juice, Worcestershire sauce, celery salt, paprika, garlic, and pepper; blend well. Sprinkle chicken with salt, and coat with sour-cream mixture. Cover; refrigerate for at least twelve hours. Remove chicken from refrigerator, and coat with bread crumbs. Place in a single layer in a lightly greased 13" × 9" × 2" baking dish. Combine butter and shortening. Pour half of mixture over

110

chicken. Bake at 350° for forty-five minutes. Pour remainder of butter mixture over chicken, and continue to bake for fifteen minutes. Serves up to ten.

One of the truly great tight ends, **Billy Joe Dupree** is one tough man to bring down in the secondary. His corn pudding, on the other hand, will go down real easy.

## BILLY JOE'S CORN PUDDING

2 cups fresh corn, cut from cob
2 tsps. sugar
1½ tsps. salt
⅛ tsp. pepper
3 eggs, lightly beaten
1 tbsp. butter or margarine
2 cups milk

Preheat oven to 350°. Combine the corn, sugar, salt, and pepper in a bowl. Add the eggs; mix well. In a saucepan, add the butter to the milk and heat until butter is melted. Blend with corn mixture. Turn into a greased one quart casserole. Place in a pan of hot water. Bake for one hour or until a knife inserted in the center comes out clean. Garnish with fresh parsley. Serves six.

Big **John Dutton** is the defensive tackle that makes the Flex Defense inflexible to run against up the middle. In order to be able to keep on taking that beating on the outside, he is careful about what he puts inside. Here are two super-healthy favorites.

## DUTTON'S DELIGHT

1 cup pineapple
1 cup apple
2 bananas
8 whole strawberries, frozen or fresh

1 cup low-fat plain yogurt
a touch of lemon
1 tbsp. wheat germ

Blend first four ingredients in blender and stir in yogurt, lemon, and wheat germ.

Option: Increase above recipe by adding two cans thawed orange juice concentrate. Place mixture in small paper cups with wooden sticks and freeze for popsicles.

## BANANA BREAD

1 cup whole wheat flour
½ tsp. salt
½ tsp. soda
2 tsps. baking powder
⅔ cup nonfat dry milk
1 cup flour, sifted
⅓ cup wheat germ
½ cup brown sugar, packed
¼ cup walnuts, chopped
*2 medium bananas, mashed
½ cup unsalted dry roasted peanuts, chopped
½ cup raisins
3 eggs
½ cup vegetable oil
½ cup molasses
¾ cup orange juice
⅓ cup dried apricots, chopped

Combine dry ingredients, nuts, and raisins. Whirl eggs in blender until foamy. Add oil, molasses, orange juice, and bananas, whirling after each. Add apricots. Pour mixture into bowl with dry ingredients. Stir just until flour is moistened. Pour into two loaf pans and bake for one hour at 325° oven. Cool in pan slightly, remove and cool completely. When cool, wrap tightly and store overnight.

*You may substitute apples, carrots, applesauce, peaches, pears, or zucchini instead of bananas.

One of football's premier wide receivers, **Tony Hill,** is part of a tradition of great Stanford University split ends. His incredible speed is helped by this light carbohydrate concoction.

## TONY HILL'S STUFFED POTATOES

2 large potatoes
¼ cup plain yogurt
1 tbsp. skim milk
2 tbsps. chives, snipped
1 tsp. salt
⅛ tsp. garlic powder
dash pepper
2 tbsps. Parmesan cheese, grated
paprika

Scrub potatoes; prick with a fork. Bake in a 375° oven for seventy minutes or until done. Slice potatoes in half lengthwise. Scoop out inside, leaving shells intact. Mash potatoes. Add yogurt, milk, chives, salt, garlic powder, and pepper. Beat till fluffy. Spoon the potato mixture into each potato shell. Sprinkle top with cheese and paprika. Return to oven. Bake for ten minutes or until heated through. If desired, place under broiler to lightly brown tops. Makes four servings (seventy calories per serving).

**Ed Jones** may be Too Tall, but with this soup in him, he is assured of not being Too Slow.

## ED JONES'S SPANISH BEAN SOUP

2 cups dry pinto beans
6 cups boiling water
2 tsps. chili powder
2 tbsps. safflower oil
2 cloves garlic, chopped
2 onions, chopped
1 green pepper, chopped

Add pinto beans to the water. Cover and cook until almost tender (two to three hours). Add chili powder. Sauté remaining ingredients in the oil and add to beans. Simmer until everything is tender.

The Cowboys' Mr. Clutch, **Drew Pearson** always seems to be in an opening in the secondary when it counts. He'll also find his way to the table when this spicy specialty is served.

### DREW'S MEXICAN CORN BREAD

1 cup whole wheat flour
1 cup stone ground cornmeal
3 rounded tsps. baking powder
½ tsp. sea salt
1 tsp. chili powder
2 eggs, beaten
½ cup milk
½ cup safflower oil
¼ cup onion, finely chopped
¼ cup green pepper, finely chopped
2 jalapeño peppers, finely chopped

Stir the flour, cornmeal, baking powder, salt, and chili powder together in a large bowl. Add the eggs, milk, oil, onion, and peppers. Beat all ingredients together (about one minute). Pour into a greased 8" × 8" pan. Bake about twenty minutes in 425° oven.

**Tom Landry** *is* the Dallas Cowboys. The only Head Coach the team has ever had, he was first an All-Pro in the secondary of the New York Giants in their glory days in the 1950's. A typical Landry creation, this bread has all sorts of variations (cornmeal instead of millet, white flour instead of wheat, etc.).

### LANDRY'S EZEKIEL BREAD
### (EZEKIEL 4:9)

Approximately 7 cups whole wheat flour
(or use some unbleached white for more general appeal)

1 cup rye flour
¼ cup millet, ground (if unavailable, use cornmeal)
3 cups (or 4) bean mix (see below)
3 cups water
⅓ cup honey or brown sugar
2 tsps. salt
2 packages yeast
¼ cup oil

Bean Mix
1 cup each: barley, pinto beans, white navy beans, lentils
Cook in a pot with water until very soft, using only enough water to cook; cook for two hours. Do not boil and drain. Use mixture to blend when done. May be slightly lumpy; gives texture to bread. Freeze any that's left over for the next batch of bread.

This bread is simple to make, like any other yeast bread. You can't fail. Just be sure your yeast is dated at least three months ahead.

Take one-half cup warm water and dissolve with two packages yeast and one teaspoon sugar. Mix the remaining ingredients (except for the whole wheat and/or white flour); you will have to use your hands. Then begin to add whole wheat (and white, if you prefer) flour to this mixture until it gets dry enough for you to handle. It should still be a little sticky. Knead for a few minutes. Brush with oil in the bowl. Cover; let rise in a warm place for approximately two hours or until double in size. When doubled, punch down, and make into two long loaves, or two bread pans, greased, make nice slicing bread, or you can make them into small, individual, bulky rolls. Use your imagination! Allow to rise, uncovered, for approximately forty minutes. Cook at 350° for approximately fifty minutes or until slightly browned. Each oven varies. When done, the bread will sound hollow when tapped on the bottom.

# CHAPTER FIVE

# Basketball

Basketball is the universal American sport. It is played indoors and out, summer and winter, and in city playgrounds, suburban driveways and country backyards, plus gyms everywhere. The only knock on basketball today is that it has become a game controlled by giants. When George Mikan became the first really dominating center, six foot six was a great height for a National Basketball Association forward or center. Now it isn't exceptional for a NBA guard. What is really remarkable though is the incredible quickness and agility of these big men.

Great basketball is like ballet performed by behemoths—the clash under the boards, a quick outlet pass leading to a fast break two-on-one, a feint, a bounce pass beyond the reach of the over-extended lone defender, finally a graceful lay-up. It combines the body control of gymnastics, the sprinting and high jumping of track, the passing offense and defense of football (and occasionally the line play), and the hand-to-eye coordination of pitching. To watch Dr. J defy the laws of gravity and physiology is to see poetry in motion. And the rare individuals who possess these skills must still learn to mesh into a team.

The players that achieve greatness in basketball almost certainly could play well in almost any sport. It is no wonder then that, as a group, they are far and away the highest paid athletes in the world. Admittedly, throwing hundreds of thousands of dollars at a kid who may not have had two bits to his name can create temptation to break training. Yet, once again, the great

players who do it again and again over the years, like John
Havlicek and Willis Reed, apply the same discipline to their
lifestyles as they do to their games. Here are their, and other
stars, thoughts on nutrition, plus those of L.A. Head Coach Pat
Riley and some do's and don'ts from Al Domenico, trainer of the
Philadelphia 76ers.

As Dr. J exemplifies the "small" forward, **Maurice Lucas** of
the Phoenix Suns is every coach's dream of a power forward. At
six feet, nine inches, he's tall enough to shoot and rebound
among the big boys under the basket and at 218 pounds, no one
is going to force him outside. What makes it all click is his great
shooting touch and constant drive. But what puts the power in
this forward is not red meat. "I discovered I could live without it ten years ago when I was on a tour of Russia and
Czechoslovakia. I didn't have any meat and I found that I didn't
miss it."

In redesigning his diet, Lucas consulted Dick Gregory, the
comedian and social activist who had previously helped
Muhammad Ali. The forward tried vegetarianism, but it left
him without sufficient energy, so he added chicken and fish. "I
find I play better on light, easy to digest foods—light proteins,
fruit, vegetables, and fresh vegetable juices plus my staple carbohydrates, spaghetti and brown rice. Breakfast the day of a
game will be enormous; toast, eggs, and oatmeal with butter and
honey. Lunch, eaten three or four hours before a game, might
consist of a tuna-fish sandwich and fresh orange juice. After the
game, a light dinner of a salad and grilled chicken is all that I
want."

With his talent, basketball is easy. What bothers him, though,
is all the traveling. "I've overcome the stress by doing as the
Romans did. I try to make the time adjustment as quickly as
possible and follow it. I'll eat dinner at the local dinnertime,
even if it's three hours off from my home."

Lucas applies that same thoughtful attitude to his overall
view of the importance of a careful diet: "An athlete's livelihood
depends on his health. The high-paced life of a professional
athlete makes him more aware of his body, which he can no
longer take for granted."

Few people look down on Lucas. One of them is **Marvin "The**

117

Human Eraser" Webster. A *really* big man, Webster has been rejecting everything that came his way on two coasts, first with the Seattle Supersonics then the New York Knicks. His basketball ways haven't changed, but like Lucas, his dietary ideas have, although his reasons are different.

"I used to eat a lot of junk food," he confesses. "Then when I became ill a few years ago I learned that proper diet is essential for everyone's well-being." As a result, breakfast now will be either his own special drink—protein powder blended with pineapple juice, bananas, strawberries, and some honey—or eggs with whole wheat toast, a fresh glass of orange juice, and some bacon. With breakfast he always takes his vitamins, usually a multiple plus additional B complex, C, and E along with calcium.

"On a game day, I have a large lunch and I feel that I have more energy on steak." With this he'll have vegetables and a glass of freshly squeezed orange juice. Also, whenever he can get them, Marvin likes fresh vegetable juices, usually carrot, sometimes carrot mixed with celery. One hour before a game he'll take some more vitamin C and will also have another glass of orange juice. Then its orange juice once again after the game.

Dinner is usually light. Even on the road Webster says you can always find a seafood or a health-food restaurant. "The league tries to book us into hotels that are near a restaurant that is open late. Even if it is just a fast food place, usually it's still possible to eat well. More and more of those places are offering salad bars, and you almost always can get something like a sandwich."

Off-season, Webster eats less red meat and stays with fish and poultry. Instead of three large meals, he finds it more comfortable to eat four or five small meals a day. If he's eaten a substantial lunch, his favorite dinner is a large vegetable platter of broccoli, asparagus, spinach, and carrots "cooked in a wok, Chinese style." His dessert will be fruit—a mixture of bananas, plums, grapes, mangoes, and papaya. He drinks only herbal teas and snacks on fresh fruit. Does all this work? Webster thinks so: "Being on a sound nutritional program made an incredible difference in my health. I could never go back to eating the way I did."

Webster's most illustrious predecessor in the pivot for the

Knicks was the Captain, **Willis Reed.** His brilliant career started as a monstrous power forward, one of the first, but came into full bloom as the imposing center for the NBA Championship team. No Knick fan (and few Laker fans) will ever forget Reed's inspiring entrance and quick two baskets over Wilt Chamberlain that provided the boost in the Knicks victory in the final game of the 1970 NBA Championships, in spite of the serious knee injury that kept him out of the rest of the game.

Now the Head Coach at Creighton University, Reed is still very much in the game. "Basketball is a demanding sport; players have to be in top physical condition at all times. Over the years I have become more aware of proper diet, more conscious of the values of certain foods, and I know that my players have, too. For example, red meat is being replaced more and more by chicken, fish, salads, and steamed vegetables. The two things that I advise are to get enough sleep and eat regularly and healthfully. For a quick booster snack, I recommend orange juice—which is what the team drinks during quarters. This goes right to the bloodstream and is a terrific energy giver."

When he's not on or by the court, Reed's hobby is great for good eating. "I have my own fishing boat, and my favorite sport is catching striped bass. Nothing's better than fresh bass. It's delicious steamed with vegetables like carrots, celery, and squash, but the following is my favorite recipe":

### WILLIS REED'S STRIPED BASS

One whole striped bass (about 3 ½ lbs.), eviscerated and cleaned
2 tbsps. fresh rosemary leaves
2 cloves garlic, minced
2 tsps. coarse salt
1 tsp. freshly ground pepper
½ lemon.

Preheat the oven to 375°. Wash the fish and dry it with paper towels. Roll out a large sheet of heavy duty aluminum foil, shiny side up. Sprinkle the center with about one quarter of the garlic, rosemary, salt,

119

and pepper. Place the fish across the center of the foil. Sprinkle the inside of the bass with half the rosemary, garlic, salt and pepper. Squeeze about half the juice from the lemon over the cavity. Close the fish and sprinkle the remaining seasonings over the top. Squeeze more lemon juice over the fish. Close the foil tightly over the fish, turning up the ends to prevent leakage. Place in a baking pan in the oven for twenty minutes. Carefully turn the package over and bake for fifteen more minutes. Remove from the oven and let it cool for ten minutes without unwrapping. Unwrap and serve. Serves four.

The sparkplug of those great Knick teams was unquestionably **Walt "Clyde" Frazier.** His quick hands made him as much a terror on defense as offense. I first asked Frazier about his diet back in his playing days. This is what he said:

"I've discovered what is good for me by a process of trial and error. Every day I take a tablespoon of cod-liver and wheat-germ oil, plus vitamin C and brewers' yeast. I eat fruit and vegetables, organically raised chicken and turkey, but hardly any red meat. Breakfast is usually steel-cut oatmeal. Before a game I'll have something like steamed spinach with brown rice and sesame seeds washed down with a glass of carrot, spinach, and celery juice. I also do yoga.

"Does my regime work? Well, look at the other guys, then look at me!"

**John "Hondo" Havlicek** is one of the few contemporaries of Frazier who could stand the comparison. The Bouncin' Buckeye ranks among the all-time greats of the Boston Celtics, therefore the NBA. First famous as their sixth man, Havlicek was a star at forward and occasionally as a guard. Relentless defense, constant effort and movement and an unstoppable jump shot made him the perfect team player.

Havlicek is as serious about his diet as his defense: "While I was playing I would eat large breakfasts consisting of orange, grapefruit, or cranberry juice, bacon and eggs, or bananas sliced on cold cereal plus whole wheat toast, hot tea or milk, and always melon if it was available—cantaloupe, musk melon, or honeydew. For a pregame meal, which I would eat at two-thirty, I went for years thinking that steak, salad, and a baked potato were the things to eat before a game. Now of course there is a lot more emphasis on pasta and lighter proteins such as chicken. Many of the players eat tuna fish and noodles, or chicken and noodles, sometimes with rice. Potatoes at least are still good. After a game I would have Italian food; veal, pasta, vegetables, and a salad. I am not a big pie and cake eater. I would rather have another pork chop than anything sweet.

"It always bothered me back then to see people in the locker room eating popcorn or drinking soda right before the game. I was extremely disciplined. I ate six hours before the game and felt that feeling slightly hungry will make you less sluggish.

"I have another secret," Havlicek continued. "When I was in training camp at the start of the season I would always report to the camp a couple of pounds *underweight*. My normal playing weight was 205 to 208, but I would go in to camp at 192. That way, when I really needed to eat a lot for energy, I wouldn't have to starve to lose the pounds I put on over the summer. The ones who have to lose were miserable. Here they worked all morning and all afternoon and had to diet on top of it. I worked hard, but I was also able to eat—big breakfasts, big lunches, big dinners, and snacks as well. If you work out, you should be able to eat more.

"Now, of course, my life is completely different. When you're playing you're not allowed to do lots of things, like skiing. So I've made up for lost time. You've heard of a bogey golfer. You might say I'm a bogey everything—fishing, tennis, white-water rafting, canoeing, you name it. My diet has changed as well. I don't need as much fuel so I eat less. Breakfast is juice and then one egg instead of two. During the day I nibble on fresh fruit. Lunch is a sandwich and dinner is generally some protein, vegetables, and a salad.

"We try to encourage our children into proper nutrition as well. For example, when they get home from school instead of eating potato chips or candy, they find a platter of cut up vegetables: usually peppers, cauliflower, broccoli, and celery. Sometimes they'll eat them plain, at times we add an onion dip."

Is nutrition important? "Well, let me tell you a story. Back in 1974, it was one day away from the end of the season, we had just played a double overtime game and I was exhausted. The fatigue was in every pore, but the next day we had to go to Milwaukee for the seventh and final game of the NBA Championships. My first reaction was to crawl into bed after the game and sleep until the next morning, but I knew that I had to give my body some fuel otherwise it never would be able to perform the next day. I remember going to a restaurant and literally forcing myself to eat—it took three and a half hours! I seem to remember it being steak and pasta, with a shrimp cocktail to start."

Suffice it to say, I am happy to report, that the next day Havlicek felt a lot better and was able to lead the Celtics to victory.

The star of that Milwaukee team in 1974 was the man who has dominated the NBA for over ten years—**Kareem Abdul-Jabbar.** Abdul-Jabbar's sky hook has brought a basket of titles since then to the Los Angeles Lakers. And while opponents' fingers and elbows made him resort to using goggles, the only thing that used to really trouble him was repeated bouts with migraine headaches and energy losses.

Abdul-Jabbar had seen numerous physicians and therapists over the years, with no results. Recently, he took his problems to Dr. Robert Giller in New York, who prescribed a cytotoxic food allergy test, to see if the cause was hidden food allergies. Abdul-Jabbar was asked to fast overnight, and the next morning one test tube of blood was taken. The results of the test are based on observing under a microscope the reactions between living white blood cells and food allergens. White blood cells are destroyed if specific antibodies to food are present.

Abdul-Jabbar was diagnosed as having allergies to wheat, eggplant, tomatoes, monosodium glutamate, milk, and shellfish. The doctor's recommendations to him were (1) to eat well-balanced meals at regular intervals, (2) to avoid, in addition to the things he is allergic to, sugar and other sweets, coffee and tea, (3) to decrease the amount of fat in the diet, and (4) to add more fresh vegetables and fruit along with fish and chicken.

Abdul-Jabbar revised his diet accordingly. Eureka!

A Phi Beta Kappa superstar at the University of Maryland

and a superstar in the NBA with the Hawks and the Bullets, **Tom McMillen** is often compared to Bill Bradley. Like the Senator from New Jersey, who starred for the great Knick teams of Reed and Frazier, McMillen passed up a direct shot with the NBA to spend a year in Oxford as a Rhodes Scholar (and then a stint in Italy). And as with Dollar Bill, the break was followed by a long and successful career in the pros anyway. They differ in two ways: at six feet, ten inches, McMillen is about five inches taller, even though they played the same position, and his well-known political ambitions have *so far* remained unfulfilled.

McMillen's desires about diet, however, have been satisfied. "I used to be a fanatic about good nutrition. Now that I have developed a pretty sound diet, I try to stick to it as much as possible and after that, food doesn't really mean that much anymore. If I have a preference, I would always choose a pregame meal of fish and salad. I have to eat at one for an eight o'clock game as having anything at all in my stomach before I play just makes me ill."

McMillen has cereal, toast, and orange juice for breakfast, and his protein is fish at lunch. Dinner after a game is whatever is available although he tries to stay away from red meat. As far as eating complex carbohydrates goes, "They don't really make a difference to me. The time I ate them the most was when I lived in Italy." Hard to avoid it there.

His platform plank on nutrition: "In general, there is an incredible overconsumption factor in America. People overeat. My advice is to try to keep meals sparing."

A Rhodes Scholar might say that **Buck Williams,** the young All-Star power forward of the up and coming New Jersey Nets, is more Macbeth than Falstaff—for him sleep is more important than food. "If you get enough rest," he feels, "everything else just falls into place." Williams tries to get a two hour nap in the afternoon before every game and at least eight hours the night before he plays.

While nutrition does not play an enormous role in his lifestyle ("I love steak, french fries, sausages, barbecue, and cheeseburgers"), the six foot, eight inch, 218 pounder does exert discipline in certain areas: "I love desserts, candy, and sweets,

123

but I try to watch myself." Also in the plus column is that he doesn't smoke and likes lots of fruit—peaches, plums, bananas, and strawberries most of all. The only thing he quaffs is apple and orange juice, "nothing alcoholic, not even beer." Williams takes a multi-vitamin supplement daily and feels that three or four bee pollen tablets taken two or three hours before the game give him more energy. He is also beginning to experiment with adding more carbohydrates to his diet, pancakes for breakfast, for example, and a small dish of spaghetti with lunch. Fish and soul food are his nutritional favorites, including iron-rich collard greens and black-eyed peas.

Just in case you're all wondering in which direction basketball locker-room talk is going these days, here's an insider's tip from the Nets: "They discuss different vitamins, which ones are best for what problems. And a number of players are researching the benefits of ginseng tea, which they drink around noon." While some people expound upon the virtues of its energy giving, while calming, qualities, it is also known for producing results in other indoor sports which have nothing to do with basketball. Watch for the Nets' success both at home and on the road.

The Jazz used to be in New Orleans and their star forward **Adrian Dantley** played in Los Angeles. A move and a trade split the distance, and they joined forces in Utah where Dantley has become one of the hottest superstars in the NBA. Now playing both small forward and shooting guard for a powerhouse team, he is continuing the torrid shooting that made him the NBA's Rookie of the Year in 1977 and the Scoring Champ in 1981.

Dantley is an example of the conscientious athlete who looks at performance, not awards and statistics. Even though he was the Rookie of the Year, he wasn't satisfied: "When I was a rookie I ate cheeseburgers and french fries. The theory was that if you got enough exercise, as a pro you could eat anything. But in the long run it will catch up to you. And it did in my case. I just didn't feel I had the maximum amount of energy." Now he has definite ideas on nutrition. "During the season I feel I need meat. The bones need more repair. I will eat it lean, however, as no one needs a lot of fat. The other thing that I find helps me is complex carbohydrates, a bowl of spaghetti, for example, the night before a game. Breakfast on a game day will generally be two eggs, whole wheat toast, and a glass of fresh juice. Lunch, eaten at one-thirty, will concentrate on protein, meat or chicken, always broiled, never fried, along with vegetables such as carrots, broccoli, zucchini, or cabbage, and a salad. Right before the game I might have a banana if I'm hungry. After the game, it's really too late to eat anything heavy, so it will be a light sandwich such as tuna fish. On the road I generally have pancakes before our noon practice and a light lunch. This seems to get my time clock back in order."

Off-season, six foot, five inch, 210 pound Dantley eats almost no meat at all, focusing instead on low-fat fish dishes which he has with a salad, a baked potato, and some fruit for dessert. He likes Chinese food ("lots of good vegetables") and has been known to snack on whole wheat crackers spread with peanut butter. Both on and off-season, Dantley experiments with micronutrient supplements. "I take a bit of everything, but always a multiple and extra $B_{12}$."

Unlike most of the athletes I interviewed, rugged (six foot, seven inch, 220 pound) forward **Scott Wedman** of the Boston Celtics is almost a vegetarian. He eats no meat at all but will on occasion eat fish, cheese, and eggs. His diet is a conscious effort to eat natural, whole grain products. If that sounds effete, remember that besides being an All-Star and having passed the glorious ten thousand career points mark, Wedman has also been on the NBA All-Defensive Team.

Wedman's breakfast is sprouted whole wheat bread with some butter and his own high protein drink, a blend of a cup of milk, a banana, a whole egg, a few tablespoons of protein powder and a tablespoon of lechithin granules. If he doesn't have the drink, he might have a bowl of oatmeal or an omelette.

On a game day, lunch will be between one- and two-thirty. This will generally be either a whole grain pasta dish, pancakes, a tofu sandwich with cream of vegetable soup, or a fish sandwich with some Cheddar cheese. "I have learned that different food combinations replace meat. Beans and rice, for example, are a complete protein and if they are eaten in a good combination, they cover all the bases of nutrition."

Since Wedman only eats one main meal a day, around five-thirty he will have a piece of fruit and after the game he will eat almost nothing, perhaps just a glass of carrot juice.

"The whole idea of protein in this country is overemphasized," he feels. "There should be a greater movement toward carbohydrates generally and complex carbohydrates in particular. We consume far too much protein and sugar. I used to have a sweet tooth so I took honey. But that's not all that far away from refined sugar; it acts the same way in the body. Now, the only sweets I eat are pure maple syrup and blackstrap molasses, which has iron in it."

"I also find it is essential to listen to your body. It's definitely psychological; if you feel like you're doing a good thing for it, chances are you are. If you have a craving, listen to it, you might be lacking in something for the moment. I also take bee pollen for energy and I drink about six to seven glasses of distilled water a day to flush the lactic acids out of my system."

"Traveling is somewhat of a problem, but I can get by on fish and egg dishes. I always try to hunt up a vegetarian or natural food restaurant and there usually are one or two in the cities we play in. If not, a Japanese restaurant can always assure you of a light meal with fish and vegetables." If you're at home, though, here are two of Wedman's favorite dishes as prepared by his wife, Kimberley:

## PEANUT SPAGHETTI

*Start cooking:*
½ lb. spaghetti or whole wheat spaghetti

*Sauce:* large skillet—oil as needed
1 large onion chopped
¼–½ lb. mushrooms chopped
⅛ cup soy grits (can be purchased
     from most well-stocked health-food stores)

⅓ cup sunflower seeds
¼ cup peanuts (unsalted preferred)
1 tsp. oregano
2 tbsps. fine chopped parsley
2 lb. jar of spaghetti or marinara sauce
1 tbsp. Parmesan cheese (more to taste)

Sauté onions and mushrooms. Add soy grits, sunflower seeds, peanuts, and spices. Add sauce and Parmesan. If not liquid enough, you can add a can of tomatoes, tomato paste, tomato sauce, or more marinara, whatever you have. Serve on spaghetti with more Parmesan, a great salad, and bread.

Kimberley says: "This recipe turns the best health food skeptic around!"

## WA BURGER

*Ingredients:* ⅔ cup vegetable oil
1 small eggplant peeled and diced
1 ½ cups shredded carrots
½ lb. mushrooms finely chopped
2 medium sized green peppers
2 large onions

Sauté the above ingredients.

1 ½ cups rolled oats
½ cup wheat germ
2 tsps. salt
¼ tsp. pepper
¼ cup flour

Use half allotted oil with all the ingredients to be sautéd. (A food processor will chop everything faster and give better texture.) One will need a large skillet or wok for all ingredients. Stir and turn until everything is brown and slightly cooked.

Add the oats and flour to desired consistency. When everything is mixed together, shape into patties and fry up with a little more oil or butter. They should brown on each side easily. Kimberley's comments: "They are usually moist and not quite as solid as hamburgers. But if you're a vegetarian or just curious, if you make these up just like your favorite hamburger they will be delicious."

**Pat Riley,** the coach and former star of the L.A. Lakers, has now studied the demands of NBA basketball from the vantage points on and beside the court. His analysis: "Professional basketball players are in such great shape from running up and down the court that they can eat almost anything and burn it up immediately. Nevertheless, I feel that things like too much sugar and caffeine are not advisable. Other than that, the players seem to know their bodies and how they react to certain things.

"When I was playing, the big things used to be steak, salad, tea, and toast. Now all the players are talking about pasta. These burn up quickly in the course of action. My advice for younger players is to seek out the advice of a good nutritionist."

**Al Domenico,** trainer of the NBA Champion Philadelphia 76ers, is the kind of guy Riley may have had in mind. Besides tending to sore joints (Domenico got more ink during the 1983 Playoffs for his updates on Moses Malone's knees, Andrew Toney's thigh, etc., than the players did), he takes charge of their weight training and diets. "We are in the process of getting together a list of ten commandments for basketball players. So far we only have one: 'You can't be physically fit without being healthy, but you can be healthy without being physically fit.' (In other words, everyone can ride a bike or walk to the store, but playing in the NBA is something else again.)

"My job is much easier today than it was years ago. Presently, a top athlete that is on a pro team will never let himself get out of shape. Athletes now are fine tuned and physically fit. At one time during the off-season they fell apart. Now they don't even fluctuate that much in weight. I take a player's best playing weight toward the end of the season, around February or March, and he must report to the training camp at this weight. Most top athletes know what weight they play best at; they also know that if they're overweight all they'll do is hurt themselves.

"Of course, for each athlete nutrition is a very personal thing. I'm not saying that all of them go home and whip up a salad of mung beans and lettuce. But I think if you are in tune with yourself, you know exactly what you want, and in some cases, what you want would make every trainer and health food nutritionist cringe. Take, for example, Maurice Cheeks, a great All-Star guard with tremendous speed. What does he live on? Something I certainly don't advocate, chocolate chip cookies and Coca Colas. And Wilt Chamberlain used to drink four quarts of Seven-Up before a game. No one has ever heard of that! Drinking carbonated soda is supposed to give you gas, at the least. But if you didn't have it for him, he wouldn't even go out on the court. So you see, players are not gods, they are just humans like you or I. They just have a need to take care of themselves and most of them do follow a pretty good dietary regime."

When the athletes arrive at the 76er training camp they are fined one hundred dollars for every pound they are overweight. Domenico immediately goes to work and puts them on a high protein, low carbohydrate diet. This is a quick weight loss regime consisting of a glass of juice for breakfast, and just a steak and a salad for both lunch and dinner. "Couple this with an intense workout two hours in the morning and two hours in the afternoon and these guys can knock off ten pounds in about two days. All we have to do is take them off carbohydrates and the weight will fall off."

According to Domenico, basketball requires no special diets, just a sound and balanced program to keep the players at their fittest. "You must remember that the players play for up to forty-eight minutes each game. If there is no action the clock stops. They are literally running for four hours each day. What is so phenomenal is that their pulse rates average from forty-five to fifty-five. In fact, some pulses are so low that if one of the players had a problem and he went to see a doctor, the physician might think he was having a coronary. That is perhaps the definition of being in perfect shape."

While Domenico does not recommend an across-the-board diet for all basketball players, there are certain rules and regulations that he recommends his players follow in order to remain in optimum shape.

# Al Domenico's Laws of Basketball Nutrition

1. It is important to drink significant amounts of liquids both before and after a game. After a game, of course, is when you should replenish yourself and make up for all the liquid lost in sweating. It is here I recommend water, at least seven glasses or, surprisingly enough, beer. A beer or two will supply the salt and minerals that are lost in the workout. The very worst thing anyone can drink after the game is soda. It is deadly. You should not replenish a tired body with sugar. It just puts a sudden surge of energy into your system and due to the rise, followed by an inevitable fall, the player becomes both irritable and lethargic, and cramps and indigestion will most likely occur.

2. Carbohydrates should be a very important part of your diet (unless you want to lose weight, then the quick weight loss diet I recommended above should be followed, but only for a day or two). Carbohydrates are more effective in the forms of bread and cereal, grain and pasta. A top player like Bobby Jones, who is one of the best defensive players ever, swears by pasta. He's an epileptic and has a special situation, but three or four hours before a game he will load up on pasta and says it works wonders for his stamina and energy. Our big, young power forward Mark Iavaroni is another athlete who is devoted to it. In fact, there is a new wave of thinking for today's athlete. Most of them are leaning toward carbohydrates, getting away from the heavy protein syndrome, and certainly cutting down on the fat, sugar, and the junk.

3. On the subject of protein. Athletes are learning more and more that energy has nothing to do with protein. In fact, a top athlete needs about the same amount of protein as a bank teller. Basketball players are usually structurally strong and there is a need for it for their muscle tissue, but not more than average.

4 and 5. Vitamins and minerals. These are not a direct source of energy, but they have a lot to do with coordinating everything in the body. I generally put my players on a vitamin program that I found works the best. Vitamin C in large doses is extremely important. The players take up to thirty-

five hundred mgs a day (about seven capsules). I feel that vitamin C maintains your well-being and keeps you healthy. Also, it helps your muscles to heal a lot faster. If you are a smoker or a drinker (most of the players are neither) then it is especially valuable to take vitamin C, as those things deplete the body's supply. Besides, what you don't need your body gets rid of anyway. I also recommend a multi-vitamin and mineral tablet along with extra A, B complex, D, and E.

All players should be sure that their diets have representatives of the following four groups every day:

1. Fruits and vegetables (carbohydrates, vitamins, and minerals).
2. Cereals and grains (again carbohydrates plus other vitamins and minerals).
3. High quality protein.
4. Milk and milk products.

Couple this every day with a decent amount of exercise and you'll always be in great shape. Athletes will just take larger portions of everything than what is needed by the average person.

In summary, in the 1960's the only foods that most athletes thought about were cheeseburgers, hamburgers, and beers. All that has changed. The only problem is, of course, when they're traveling. When we get through with a game at eleven-thirty or midnight there are very few restaurants open, only junk food places. But even then, most of the players are finding ways of getting around that. Does it work? Well look at Dr. J. He's a superb athlete and he makes sure that he takes care of himself every day of the year. He is already tuned into conditioning, but he will still listen to and try new ideas and suggestions, and let you know what he thinks. He is what I like all my players to be, conscientious about his weight. In fact, he never varies more than a few pounds from one season to the next. These players are getting paid to stay in good shape. If there is one across-the-board suggestion I would have, it's don't overindulge in anything!

# CHAPTER SIX

---

# Hockey

The joy of watching a Gretzky or Bossy leave opponents poke-checking at empty ice to blast a radar guided missile into the back of the net to break a tie with seconds left on the clock ranks right up there with other great sports moments. A Jackson home run in the bottom of the ninth, an Abdul-Jabbar slam dunk at the buzzer or Clark catching a TD bomb off a hopeless scramble with no time left has nothing on them.

But unlike those other fellows, hockey players never play more than one or two minutes at a time. The demands of hockey on the system are so intense that even the finest athletes exhaust their available blood sugar, and it and they need to be constantly replaced. Their bodies need to break down the glycogen in the muscles, replenish the blood sugar flow, and remove the lactic acid—then go out and sprint again. Hockey is the antithesis of a game like soccer where substitution is almost a crime, and baseball where when you're out you're gone. But in no other sport is the opportunity for rest during the flow of the game so infrequent. After all, when you go out of bounds in football the play stops. In hockey you just bounce off the sideboards.

Of course, the nutritional guidelines discussed in Chapter 2 can be critical to avert cramping and fatigue while playing a dynamic winter sport in varying climates. It is therefore no surprise that today's top hockey stars share the diet consciousness of their football counterparts.

The coming of age of nutritional awareness in hockey is best described by the man who epitomizes the game. At the top of everyone's All-Time list is **Gordie Howe.** Over thirty years in the National Hockey League, World Hockey Association and back again in the NHL, finally retiring in 1981 at the impossible age of fifty-one, Howe is the Babe Ruth of hockey. Combining scoring with tremendous upper-body strength and toughness, he was a legend in his own time.

"Years ago players thought that steak should be the main source of energy, so they ate it at three o'clock in the afternoon. I preferred to eat it at 9:00 A.M. and have eggs and pancakes in the afternoon. But we used to practice at ten o'clock in the morning so it was impossible to eat any breakfast, just a glass of orange juice and then lunch after practice. So I found that eating ground beef at noon was good because if you're excited about the game and don't chew the food as well, ground beef is more easily digested. If I was tired, I'd have a chocolate bar before the game. We never got out of the dressing room until after 1:00 A.M. and then you'd have to eat at whatever was open. By then you were usually so tired you'd eat anything. It was really a challenge to stay fit."

The rest of the players finally caught up to Howe if not on the ice at least at the table. "Now the players are going to starches and carbohydrates. I lasted thirty years without them, so I didn't change my eating habits recently. I just tended to eat meat the night before the game, although now they are saying that meat is not as good as we thought at any time. In any case, I always had a lot of energy. In fact, at fifty, I cried for more ice time."

Howe feels that weight is the most important thing in longevity. "If you are too heavy or too light you don't play well. I was 204 when I started at sixteen and 206 when I retired. I owe a lot of my success to my wife, who made sure that my meals were balanced. She always insisted on a green and yellow vegetable, salads plus a variety of different proteins, not always red meats, and fruit. Balance is important. In fact, in our brain we have the appestat which monitors the intake of food. If we are short a nutrient, we send out impulses to eat. However, if our diet is balanced and the body needs energy it goes right to breaking down the body fat, not to the lean tissue. It's the only way to really stay in top condition." Thirty years of hockey players found out in the corners that the answer to the question "Who is in the best shape?" was usually Howe.

As great as Howe's career was in the 1950's, 1960's, and 1970's, the 1980's have seen the emergence of a player whose abilities make superlatives seem ordinary. In fact his nickname is one—**Wayne "The Great" Gretzky.** His record shatterings have been by such a huge margin over those previously on the books that the only comparison that comes readily to mind is Bob Beamon's long jump in the 1968 Olympics in Mexico City. Except Gretzky didn't perform his feat once, but over and over again. While miraculous leaps may happen almost by chance, scoring over ninety goals and two hundred points in a National Hockey League season is no fluke. His latest greatest, fifty-one straight games with at least one point scored, beat the old record by twenty-one—and he had set that! Surely Gretzky's phenomenal talents are the products of not just nurture but nature, however he ascribes great importance to nutrition. "Diet is of utmost importance to a pro hockey player, especially because the seasons are as long as they are. I have always tried to eat well, but now I am learning how much more difficult it is to play up to one's potential without having eaten properly in advance." At six feet and 170 pounds, Gretzky does not have to worry about a weight-control diet, only one that is nutritionally well balanced. He eats a lot, because he feels he burns it off. In fact, Gretzky eats much more than some athletes almost twice his size, like Anthony Munoz and Too Tall Jones.

Gretzky's breakfast sounds like that of the players who eat only one meal a day: four or five scrambled eggs with bacon, whole wheat toast, and some coffee with a dash of cream, no sugar. He eats at nine and then goes off to a ten o'clock practice which lasts about forty-five minutes. At one o'clock, it's lunchtime, another feast. Gretzky will probably have a steak (his favorite) or veal, along with vegetables and a salad, and usually dessert as well. One key may be that after lunch he takes a long

134

nap, not waking up until about five o'clock, in time to go out to the arena. Presumably, this enables his body to digest breakfast and lunch.

What Gretzky does next goes against all the rules now prevalent for the diet of an athlete. Whereas most of the stars cannot even think about food before the game, Gretzky cannot think of anything *but* his stomach. Right before the game he'll have something like a grilled cheese sandwich with a large milk shake or a monte crisco (melted cheese and ham) sandwich. He might even have a piece of pie for "dessert." Obviously not one to go to sleep empty, after the game he has his last meal of the day, usually just a sandwich.

To all the self-deniers and starvers, The Great Gretzky's diet sounds outrageous. Nevertheless, it is not too far from the eating habits of another sports speedster, Rickey Henderson. Metabolic rate is the apparent answer, one with which Gretzky agrees. "My weight does not change dramatically throughout the calendar year. I'm fortunate to have a metabolism which allows me to eat whenever I want and whatever I want without gaining weight. It's the quality and the quantity that counts."

Gretzky also keeps this philosophy on travel days. He feels that the most important way to cope with the time change is to have a good breakfast to start out the day. He will always have his scrambled eggs, toast, and bacon, and will add orange juice whenever he's on the road. "The two most important bits of advice I can offer to youngsters are the following: Be sure to have a balanced diet to form the proper foundations and also get enough sleep." And you too will be able to score one hundred goals.

The New York Islanders have made history by capturing the Stanley Cup four years in a row. The captain of all those teams, and one of hockey's premier defensemen, **Denis Potvin,** is a thoughtful and articulate exponent of a carefully planned diet. In fact, Potvin has developed separate in-season and off-season regimes of diet and conditioning. "I have tried to tailor my program to the particular needs of a professional hockey player. Vegetarianism might be fine for people in less aggressive sports, but when I need brute strength I'll eat a rare steak." The rest of the time he avoids red meat and finds that chicken or fish, fruit, vegetables, and potatoes or spaghetti are all he needs for a well-rounded diet, with a premium on buying everything fresh every day. For extra energy he takes a high potency multiple vitamin capsule daily along with additional vitamins C and E and Busy Bee B complex, though he recognizes that eating properly probably makes taking large doses of vitamins unnecessary. Potvin also realizes that because hockey requires unusually large bursts of energy and exertion, muscle cramps are a potential problem. "To deal with this, I eat a lot of bananas and oranges which are high in potassium."

Potvin starts his day with fresh fruit and cereal. Lunch, his largest meal, is taken about one o'clock in the afternoon, and is based on starch (potatoes or spaghetti) before a game, poultry and fish on a nongame day. Dinner is usually light, mostly just vegetables and fruit. "If I eat a lot the night before, I can't sleep and I feel awful the next day." Although the game requires him to travel, he tries to stay on his New York time schedule. This includes, without fail, an hour and a half nap each day. Off-season he keeps in shape by jogging, playing handball and racquetball, riding a bicycle, and "cutting out the beer."

American-born and -raised players are rare enough in the NHL, but the Rangers' **Nick Fotiu** takes it one step further. Not from such snowy climes as Minnesota and New England, Fotiu is a native of New York City, Staten Island to be precise. True to his New York heritage, he loves ethnic food. Fotiu is a combination of Italian and Greek and likes the best things from both nationalities. From the Greeks comes a love of lamb's head (that he gets from his godfather's farm); the Italian side gives him a love of spaghetti, fresh clams, mussels, and squid. Fotiu likes to eat—as witnessed by his six feet, two inch, 210-pound physique, although ideally, he admits, he plays better at 213. He has never had a weight problem and he loves most food as long as it is fresh and wholesome. "I just don't eat junk food at all." He takes vitamins, though, including B

136

complex (for stress) and finds that if he's really tired, a tea-spoon of honey seems to help.

On a nongame day, Fotiu will have a very big breakfast that starts the day off right. It consists of a large glass of freshly squeezed orange juice, eggs, bacon, and sometimes pancakes or a cooked whole grain cereal like oatmeal or cream of rice. Nongame day lunches consist of a sandwich on whole grain bread or broiled fish or even a homemade pizza with just a "little tomato sauce and some freshly grated mozzarella and Parmesan." On a game day his breakfast will be much smaller. "Maybe one boiled egg, maybe nothing at all. I wait for lunch to have the meal that will give me energy to play. Spaghetti with Parmesan cheese, three eggs, and some bacon usually does it. I tend to eat a lot of spaghetti as I feel that carbohydrates give me more energy." After the game (or earlier on a nongame day) is when he will truly enjoy what he eats. Italian is the way he likes to go then, and he might begin with some fresh bean soup, followed by pasta with a thick piece of Italian bread, or fish, clams, mussels, or shrimp. He also likes veal and chicken. He'll have this with a large salad of mixed lettuce and tomatoes, and always a fresh vegetable, preferably spinach, beets, cauliflower, asparagus, or one of his specialties—broccoli rab, made by sautéing a little garlic in some olive oil, adding the broccoli rab and letting it cook for a short while. Then he pours it over a plate of macaroni.

"Off-season I have a house on Cape Cod, and it is here all my food fantasies come to light." Fotiu has his own lobster boat and fishes for a fresh catch every day. "It's heaven to be able to reach into a trap and pull out an enormous lobster. I just pull off one of the claws and eat it raw." That may be carrying freshness a little far, but will do nothing to hurt Fotiu's tough-guy image on ice. Other catches include six-inch-wide oysters and all kinds of saltwater fish. "My ideal meal out there is to have that fish (caught that morning) with a few pieces of corn on the cob and a large salad. I'm not big on desserts and I avoid chocolate at all cost."

Contrary to his image, however, Fotiu is a gourmet cook. An energy drink that he likes is made from throwing a handful of strawberries, blueberries, a banana, an egg, milk, ice cubes, and a dash of cinnamon into the blender and whipping it up. Here's another specialty:

## BAKED CLAMS À LA FOTIU

Put a little olive oil in a pan. Add chopped garlic to taste and chopped red pepper, sweet or hot. Brown. Add some chopped onions and brown lightly. Take clams out of their shells and chop them up. Take all the ingredients and put them into a large bowl. Add two raw eggs and mix together with the other ingredients. Put in Italian-seasoned bread crumbs, freshly grated Parmesan cheese, and mix all together with some freshly chopped parsley and oregano. Stuff everything back into the clam shells (make sure the mixture is moist enough). Put a tiny piece of bacon on top and broil each one until brown on top.

The best record in the 1982–83 NHL season belonged to the Boston Bruins, who many feel also have the game's best defenseman, **Brad Park,** who is now with the Detroit Red Wings. Another veteran athlete who has discovered the benefits of a planned diet, Park admits: "The older I get, the more conscious I've become of nutrition. I'm not fanatic about it, however. For example, if during the season I want to stop off and have an ice cream cone, I'll have it. I know I just burn it off during a practice. On a game day I'll eat my big meal about twelve-thirty or one o'clock; that way my stomach will be free for the game. In the morning I'll just have some fresh orange juice and an English muffin. After the late morning practice skate I will have some pasta, like spaghetti, and veal Parmesan. The night before a game I tend to eat more carbohydrates, more bread and starches. With this I will have white meat of chicken or turkey or fish. Steak used to be my favorite food, but after I moved to Boston, I found that I ate much more fish. However, in a body contact sport it is difficult to cut out red meat entirely. You tend to need the strength that it gives you, so I make a point of working it in regularly during the season. I try to have this meal at least twenty-four hours before a game as I don't like to feel full, ever. Since I don't drink much coffee at other times, I find that caffeine gives me an incredible lift. About an hour and a half before the game I will drink three or four cups of straight black coffee. Caffeine gets the blood going. I might also have a chocolate bar then. After the game, I find that three or four beers replace the fluids that I lose in each game." While this may sound unseemly, Park's system does make sense for a hockey player. Caffeine without sugar has been shown to have a stimulating effect and the fats and sugar in chocolate provide peak energy, over a longer period of time than sugar alone. The beers are needed to replace the B vitamins used in processing the chocolate and fluids lost to the diuretic action of the coffee. Needless to say, in the long run, there are a lot better ways of doing it.

Park also tailors his menu to his schedule. "If I'm not playing that day I won't eat much at all. I'll just have juice for breakfast, a salad, and a sandwich for lunch and a nice dinner with protein, salad, and vegetables." Park shares Potvin's concern about getting enough rest, but he handles it less systematically. "There is, of course, a great deal of traveling involved in hockey, and the hardest part of that is the loss of sleep. I can go for about three or four weeks without a whole lot of sleep, and then I'll just crash and sleep for two days. Actually, unlike most guys, the time that I can lose weight the easiest is when I'm on the road. There are no refrigerators in the room, and no one is there baking cookies. Also, on the road I'll make a conscious effort not to drink anything but water. Off-season I don't do very much for about two months. I'm usually worn-out from the playoffs." That's a problem a lot of other players would love to have. Six or eight weeks before camp he'll start biking, swimming, and working out on the Nautilus to prepare for the season.

"What advice do I have for youngsters? Well, I have five children (ages eleven, ten, seven, six, and three) and I feel it's best not to force kids to eat. Don't, for example, say you can only have dessert if you finish your dinner. Teach them to eat only as much as they need, and give small portions. Don't encourage them to become hearty eaters or you're just asking for them to have weight problems when they get older. I was always a chunky kid who always had two helpings of everything. That's another thing. Seconds are not allowed in my household." It sounds like Park is as good a father as he is a defenseman.

Everyone on the Islanders is dangerous (even Billy Smith, their goalie). But it doesn't take more than a second for any opponent to single out the guy they fear the most—sharpshooting wing **Mike Bossy.** And it's not because of cheap shots or fast fists, since Bossy was awarded the Lady Byng Trophy for sportsmanlike conduct for the 1982–83 season. Bossy just puts the puck in the net more than any other winger in hockey.

Bossy is the type of high performance athlete who is lean (six feet, one inch and 190 pounds) and who backs into a high octane diet. "I don't look upon food as motivation or preparation for the game. I eat because I find it necessary, and I also eat only when I'm hungry." Breakfast for Bossy during the season is simply coffee and a donut at ten-thirty. He practices for an hour and a half (the coffee and donut are burned up along the way), and then about one o'clock he will have something light, usually a sandwich and a bowl of tomato soup. A few hours before the game he will have his final pregame meal. If he's at home, its generally scrambled eggs with pancakes, or French toast. On the road, however, it is generally a steak and a baked potato. Off-season, in the morning he has toast and coffee and a variety of fresh fruit—honeydew, melon, cherries, and grapes. After that he doesn't have set mealtimes, he just picks at things. Nevertheless, his dietary predilections make a good deal of sense. "I used to be a dessert eater, but now I'm not. I have cravings and I'll eat things for about three days, then I won't have them again. My ideal dinner is roast beef, mashed potatoes with peas, and a chocolate fondue in which I dip every kind of fruit." Not exactly health food, but still a solid, sensible diet for a pro hockey player.

The best all-around hockey player today? It could well be Bossy's longstanding linemate **Bryan Trottier,** the New York Islanders' All-Star center. A superb skater, passer, shooter, and checker, Trottier is a master of every phase of the game. He is also very much in control of his diet.

Basically, Trottier feels that a good diet is essential to the life of an athlete. "If you don't watch your diet you tend to become tired and lazy and lack spunk. It is not food, in general, but the lack of it that gives the energy. One good meal a day should be sufficient. People make the mistake of getting too weighed down by food. If I start to feel tired, I'll eat less and lighter meals, and then I'll have more energy." The exception to that rule is a good steak. Trottier has found that red meat gives him strength and energy if he eats it the night before a game. "Players who only eat chicken and fish tend to lose something," he feels. "The only time I give up red meat is in the summertime, when I tend to gain a little more weight."

On a game day, Trottier will have his big meal at one o'clock in the afternoon. This will consist of a steak, baked potato, vegetable, and toast, or eggs, sausage, and toast. "Carbohydrate loading does nothing for me," he admits, "but I do feel you need a good mix of protein and carbohydrates for energy. I also vary the carbohydrates, my favorites being rice, potatoes, and spaghetti. I don't drink any alcoholic beverages, very rarely eat desserts, almost never eat chocolate and never crave junk." Basically, Trottier doesn't go overboard on anything. He has been overdoing it lately on Stanley Cups, but that is an addiction he's happy to have.

Another Stanley Cup winner with the Islanders, **Glen "Chico" Resch,** was the man the New Jersey Devils went after to build their defense around. Being the bulwark of a young team, Resch has become a very busy goaltender. Fortunately, at five feet, nine inches and 170 pounds, he has always kept himself in perfect condition.

"Consistently good nutrition plays an essential role for all athletes. Weight fluctuations of even four or five pounds can be crucial." Resch is very careful with his diet. He starts with a good pregame meal about seven hours before the game. "If you eat well, not just a lot of empty calories, it makes the difference in the second or third period when you need to feel stronger. I used to eat very lightly before a game, and then I had an energy crisis in the later periods." Breakfast on a non-game day is usually very small, just a glass of juice. "We go to practice early and I don't like to have a full stomach." After practice it's cold cereal, generally Raisin Bran, alternating with scrambled eggs and whole wheat toast. "I never eat any fried food, like bacon or sausage, and I'll have lots of fruit, my favorites being bananas, oranges, and peaches. On a game day I'll have a glass of orange juice and a piece of toast for breakfast and then will have a large lunch for the pregame meal. This will consist of a small salad, followed by macaroni or spaghetti with tomato sauce and some Parmesan cheese grated on top, along with a small hamburger or meat balls, veal or fish, plus vegetables, preferably broccoli or peas. I will never have anything heavy like a large steak as I find it much too difficult to digest. My favorite meal is to boil some macaroni, in a separate pan lightly sauté a little chopped meat with onions, mix in the noodles and sprinkle with some cheese."

For all those shooters frustrated by Resch over the years, there is a glimmer of hope—he does have a weakness. "My favorite dessert, which I know is sinful, is chocolate-marshmallow-almond ice cream. After the game, I will usually have something light, like a salad, some eggs or a small sandwich. However if I'm feeling heavy, I will not eat anything at all. As far as liquids are concerned, I drink a lot of bottled water and find that it really saves calories. It's better certainly than any kind of soda, as even diet soda makes you retain water. If I'm not playing that night I'll have a more substantial dinner (as I probably ate a light lunch of salad, soup, and a sandwich) which can be chicken and stir-fried vegetables, or spaghetti with peas and little pieces of ham chopped up in it."

Resch has a few words of advice for parents: "Most parents don't realize that they are creating problems for children in the future by giving them the wrong kinds of food. Don't be afraid to tell them no! When the child is young you're the one who's starting them out in life. Many parents assume that if they like something, their child will like it as well. That's why, for example, so many parents just slab butter and jelly on their child's bread. They assume that because they like it that way, the child will also. Parents who eat a lot themselves tend to give their children too much food. You must be careful not to pass on your bad eating habits." Chocolate-marshmallow-almond ice cream being the sole exception.

**Barry Beck,** Captain and All-Star defenseman for the New York Rangers, is one of hockey's real blocks of granite. "Nutrition plays a very important role in your performance," he feels. "I have drastically changed my diet over the years. Up until I was twenty, I ate everything. But slowly I discovered what my body reacts to—what I feel well with and the foods that don't agree with me. I find that I get a negative response from sweets, fats, and dairy products."

"On a game day I'll eat about five or six hours before we play. Then I'll have some pasta, perhaps linguini (easy on the clam sauce) and some whole grain bread. My normal diet is a breakfast of fruit, especially some melon, which contains water and is very important since our systems are about ninety percent water. For lunch I'll have a large mixed green salad with some hard boiled eggs and plain yogurt as dressing. I'll spice it up with different herbs and add tomatoes, cucumbers, carrots, and pieces of whole wheat bread. I include whatever I can find that is good and fresh. Dinner is chicken (I'll take the skin off before broiling it) or fish and a variety of vegetables, such as squash, broccoli, cauliflower, and green beans. In addition, I'll have corn on the day of the game because that contains more starch. The vegetable I love most of all, though, is onions, cooked, raw, served in any way (I always wondered why nobody gives me a hug on the ice). After the game, I find I must replace the nutrients, so I have a good steak, a salad, and some soup." Being six feet, three inches and about 205 pounds, Beck has to eat to keep up with Gretzky, at least on the ice if not at the table.

Expansion teams were the butt of a lot of jokes around the NHL until the Philadelphia Flyers took the Stanley Cup away from the old line clubs. The leader of the Broad Street Bullies then and now is **Bobby Clarke,** centerman extraordinaire. Clarke's brand of hockey is intelligent, aggressive, and nonstop effort. He is a complete player, brilliant on defense as well as offense. As one would expect, that completeness extends to his preparation for the game.

"Proper nutrition is as important to the athlete as the physical part of training. Like most athletes, I changed my ideas about six years ago when we were first made aware that it is not protein that is the main source of fuel for the body, but complex carbohydrates." On the other hand, Clarke feels that each person should experiment with food to find out what is right. No one diet or program will work for everybody, because everyone's body and metabolism is different. "You have to do it on your own. It's almost a process of trial and error. If you know that something makes you sick, you just don't eat it." Because Clarke has diabetes, he has to be especially careful about his diet.

Clarke has found that he plays well on lots of complex carbohydrates such as spaghetti, potatoes, and bread, and that not too many calories on a game day works best for him. "What is right for me I know about, but I really cannot say what will be the best for everyone else. You have to read books and get advice from a dietician as to what is right for an athlete and then the amount you take in you have to figure out for yourself. Obviously, one of the main things is to drink lots of water. Other than that, there are really no secrets."

A few years back, When the New York Rangers were looking to add a spark to their offense, they imported (at great expense) two sensational Swedish skaters by way of the old WHA. **Anders Hedberg** and Ulf Nilsson helped open up the vistas for the flying foreigners who have brought oomph to the NHL.

"I follow a normal, highly nutritious diet," says Hedberg. "We play so many games that I need the energy one has from being very fit. I couldn't make it unless I was." Breakfast consists of fresh juices, bread home-baked by his wife, Gunn-Marie, cereal (usually Corn Flakes with bananas), and tea. "Lunch, eaten at one-thirty, is my main meal, so I really consider it dinner. For that meal I will generally have something like chicken with brown rice, a salad, and a glass of milk. I like to have a variety of foods, always healthy, and

144

will sometimes have steak, liver, or fish, and instead of rice, spaghetti or fettucini, with vegetables. I do believe in eating more carbohydrates, like noodles, on a game day, but I will not eat meat then. Fish is my favorite because it is light to digest. Before a game, I will generally have a cup of coffee and a small pastry at four-thirty." After the game at eleven or eleven-thirty he doesn't eat too much, generally a bowl of soup, a salad, and an omelette. "It's better to go to sleep with an empty stomach. On a nongame day, since I've eaten my big meal for lunch, I will have a sandwich at about eight o'clock."

Hedberg says that you can lose close to a gallon of liquids during each game, so he drinks before and after the game as well as between periods. He usually drinks a special concoction from Sweden called Pripps which restores some of the electrolytes that are lost during the game. "Sleep is also important," he feels. "I need at least eight hours." Off-season he plays tennis for recreation, jogs, lifts weights, and limits his fat intake. It just proves that nutrition, like sports, is completely international.

## ANDERS HEDBERG'S WHITE BREAD

Ingredients:
6 cups flour
3 pkgs. active dry yeast (¾ oz.)
2 tsps. salt
1 cup water
1 cup 2% low-fat milk
4 tbsps. vegetable oil

Mix four cups of the flour with salt and yeast. Heat water and milk to warm, add oil and pour over flour mixture. Mix well and gradually add flour till dough is nice and smooth. Let dough rest at least fifteen minutes. Knead dough well, make two loaves, put in greased pan. Let rise till double size. Bake in 450° F oven thirty to thirty-five minutes. Keep covered while cooling.

## RYE BREAD (LINGONBERRY BREAD)

Ingredients:
4 cups rye flour
3 pkgs. yeast
1 tbsp. salt
1 oz. margarine
2 cups milk
4 oz. Swedish lingonberries
2 cups white flour

Mix three cups of the rye flour with yeast and salt. Melt margarine, add milk, heat to warm. Pour over flour mixture, mix, add lingonberries, mix well. Add the rest of the rye flour, and gradually add white flour till dough is smooth. Let rise covered until dough has doubled its size. Knead dough well. Split dough and make two round "cakes." Make lines with knife. Let rise covered till doubled size (thirty minutes). Bake in 450°F oven for ten minutes, lower to 350°, bake thirty to forty-five minutes. Keep covered while cooling.

When one of the New York Rangers feels sore, he comes to trainer **Bob Williams.** Not only does Williams strap a bad ankle or relieve a muscle ache but he is acutely aware of nutritional needs. His job is also to make sure that the players don't get injured. To that end, he believes that good diet is essential for maintaining the players in top form.

"Nutrition is a part of our lives and you should look upon it as something that can be abused like drugs or alcohol. The abuse of food can be just as detrimental to the health and well-being of athletes as to every other human being. Nutrition starts within the family. If the parents follow a good diet it produces good dietary habits in the children. I am also a firm believer in not changing things that work for you. If you have a well-balanced diet and good foundations and come from an ethnic background, you shouldn't stray too much from that diet. For example, Eddy Mio (now with Detroit) comes from an Italian background and he does very well sticking to Italian food. That diet has suited him well and he thrives on the spaghetti and other pastas and sauces. But for someone like Ron Greschner with his background in

British Columbia, to start getting into hot curries before a game would be foolish. He would only get sick.

"As for vitamins, I'm neither for or against them. Many times they give the players a psychological boost, and the body tends to rid itself of the ones that are not used. We actually provide vitamins to the players if they feel they are not eating right. In fact, I highly recommend them to our single athletes who don't know much about cooking and don't give their diets too much thought. I also think it's important to keep a diary of what you're eating. So many people just eat, and at the end of the day they have no idea how much they've consumed. For example, all athletes are invited to functions. They almost always end up standing around the hors d'oeuvres table or eating cheese and crackers. In the process, an enormous amount of calories are consumed absentmindedly.

"Above all, whether it's from the home or later on, nutrition is an educational experience. Europeans historically tend to be more conscious of a good diet. Hedberg, for example, has very good eating habits. On the other hand, Beck is an example of the new wave of North American player who is consistently becoming more and more conscious of his diet."

The following are Williams's ideas about the right diet for hockey players in any level of play:

The main meal for a contest is the one that is eaten the night before. By the time that you play, that food has been broken down and put into value by the muscles. It should be high in protein: red meat, chicken, pork, fish. Vegetarians can still get an adequate amount of proteins from certain vegetables, nuts, and seeds. This meal should be eaten about four hours before you go to sleep. An ideal menu would be:

6 to 8 ounces of roast beef, medium rare
a baked potato (eat the skin; it is high in minerals)
green vegetables—broccoli, string beans, spinach, etc.
a large green salad, with mixed lettuce, tomatoes, cucumbers, carrots, and a light vinaigrette dressing
fruit salad for dessert.

147

Instead of drinking wine, which you tend to feel the next day, or a sugary soft drink, or coffee or tea (with caffeine that will keep you up), the best drink possible is water. Try not to drink it with the meal, but after. Let your own natural digestive juices work for you without diluting them.

Breakfast on game days should serve two purposes. It should simply take away the hunger pangs and should be easily digestible, so you don't have to go on the ice with a feeling of fullness. If you decide on eggs, frying is not recommended since the grease tends to lie heavy in the stomach. No bacon or ham either for the same reason. One or two poached or boiled eggs plus carbohydrates, such as one or two pieces of whole grain toast, and a glass of freshly squeezed fruit juice is a good way to start. Bananas (for potassium) and fresh oranges are also good, or cereal with toast plus fresh fruit juice. I don't think coffee is great, but the Russians seem to believe in it and have been known to drink gallons of the stuff before a game. If you deprive your body of coffee for a week and then just have some when you need it on a certain day, the caffeine does give an extra spurt of energy. If you drink milk, make it the low-fat skim milk variety, as it is much easier to digest. This is the time to take a multi-vitamin.

Lunch should be eaten five or six hours before a contest, and should consist of easily digestible proteins, such as fish, and carbohydrates. I recommend that the meal be something like four to five ounces of fish with some noodles or pasta, staying away from meat sauce. Tuna fish is also good. The idea is to provide enough carbohydrates for energy and to fill you up but not overfill you. You should feel comfortable but somewhat hungry. This should be accompanied by plenty of water to maintain good functioning of body and muscle cells. No alcohol, but a slice or two of bread (stay away from butter or margarine) and a small salad for roughage. Dessert can be a small dish of ice cream.

About two hours before the game it's a good idea to have a few small cookies or bread sticks with lots of water. It takes a lot of energy to digest a Coke, which is full of sugar. Water is always the best. Even the electrolyte drinks have to be digested, and the blood has to go there and break it down instead of being used for other things.

After the game it is best to stick with something light.

148

Bread sticks and a salad, or crudités such as raw cauliflower and carrot sticks, with a blue-cheese dip. Lots of water, as always, or one beer. If there is something to celebrate, a glass of champagne. Finally, a little later, have a light easily digestible dinner. A small amount of fish or chicken plus a small bowl of soup would be good, as would an omelette, with fruit and yogurt for dessert. Sleep is very important that night. Try to get as much as possible.

# CHAPTER SEVEN

# Soccer

In the rest of the world besides the United States soccer (known as football every place else) is far and away the most popular team sport. Here it used to be a game only associated with ethnic urban groups. But that was in the era B.P. (Before Pelé). Now, it is clearly the fastest growing major sport among the entire cross section of American kids, from peewee to college. Soccer's attraction to parents as well as children is that it requires stamina and coordination and is a fresh air sport that can be played in most areas and weather, yet does not put a premium on physical contact or even above-average size. In fact, since it doesn't require the exceptional hand-to-eye coordination of baseball and basketball, it also permits more participation from the less than spectacularly skilled.

The grass-roots movement from youth soccer on up is eventually going to produce enough world-class U.S.-born athletes like Ricky Davis for us to take a serious run at the World Cup. The 1986 affair will tell us how far we've come to date. But in any case, the North American Soccer League, and specifically the N.Y. Cosmos, brought soccer into the major leagues of professional sports in this country when Pelé, the immortal Brazilian genius of the sport, came to New York in 1975. The additions of Italian League scoring champ Giorgio Chinaglia in 1976 and in 1977 Franz Beckenbauer, probably the greatest midfielder ever to play the game, made the Cosmos a box office draw in the U.S. and a global soccer power. Along the way they also had the best record in the North American Soccer League regular season every year from 1978 through 1983 and won the Soccer Bowl in 1977, 1978, 1980, and 1982.

The rise in soccer popularity here was evidenced by the first live network broadcast of a World Cup Championship Match in 1982. With the Olympic Games bringing top flight amateur soccer to Los Angeles, the local interest should get another major boost. It's unfortunate that the U.S. effort to host the 1986 World Cup Games foundered on the shores of international sports politics. It would have put soccer over the top in the U.S. Nevertheless, with Team America in the NASL, a strong showing is still possible. Team America is the American unit put together with a view to developing a cohesive national team for the World Cups. Even modest success in nearby Mexico should galvanize American interest.

Since widespread soccer popularity here is relatively new and basically growing along with today's health-conscious youngsters, there are no traditional hot-dog or candy-bar connotations attached to it. In addition, First Division (the name in most countries for the league including the most successful teams) level soccer is certainly as physically demanding as any of the other major professional sports, with the accent on endurance. For ninety minutes, the top stars are in constant motion up and down the field, with substitutions rarely occurring. So both homegrown and foreign soccer stars tend to be a hardy breed, devoted to good health and proper diet, albeit national predilections still play a role.

For example, some of the English players' pregame meals consist just of tea, toast, and honey. Giorgio Chinaglia, on the other hand, loves pasta and rumor has it that only his mother can cook it for him, although he won't have it on the day of the game. Whatever the diet, though, soccer requires intense energy and in all but Northern Europe is usually played in extreme heat. A player can lose an enormous amount of fluids in one afternoon and muscle cramps and heat stroke can result if proper care isn't taken. Here are the top players' secrets for keeping in excellent shape, along with advice from Striker trainer Rey Jaffet, and a diet and philosophy proposed for young soccer players and fans by Ken Schields, the trainer of the Tampa Bay Rowdies.

**Ricky Davis,** at age twenty-five, is no longer one of America's most promising young soccer players. That's because he has fulfilled that promise by becoming one of the most effective midfielders, first in the NASL with the Cosmos, and now with the St. Louis Steamers, the Major Indoor Soccer League. He may well be the best native-born American soccer player ever.

Davis became interested in nutrition through his father, a doctor. "As children, we were encouraged to develop proper eating habits," he said. "We weren't told, for example, that white bread was bad for you. We just learned that whole grain products were better. We weren't allowed to eat junk food, however, and my mother never bought it or had it in the house. If we did eat it on occasion it was an event, not a reward. Parents should take time to explain things to their children, why, for example, potato chips are not good for you, and give them good alternatives. Children should feel privileged to be able to eat wholesome food. That way they will like being in on the 'secret' and won't rebel later on."

While Davis does take a multiple vitamin, he feels that eating well makes vitamins in general unnecessary. "As athletes, the condition of our bodies is a direct factor in our ability to perform. Proper rest, good eating habits, and good practice are the best investments we can make." To that end Davis gets at least eight hours of sleep a night and makes sure he eats three balanced meals daily. He does not like to eat big breakfasts, but he begins his day with orange, apple, or tomato juice, a slice of whole grain toast, a cereal such as Grape Nuts (no sugar), and a half grapefruit. Occasionally, he will drink coffee as he feels it improves his performance, and once or twice a week he eats eggs or pancakes. Lunch will be a sandwich, usually ham, turkey, or peanut butter ("freshly ground without salt, it's high in protein and quite nutritious"), and fruit. He also likes fruit salads with nuts, especially almonds. Dinner is red meat two or three times a week, and fish or chicken the other days, with a salad, vegetables, pasta, and fruit for dessert. For a quick pickup during the day, Davis recommends drinking orange juice. Truly an All-American diet.

The man who took many of Davis's passes and puts them in the net is **Giorgio Chinaglia,** far and away the greatest scorer in NASL history. Chinaglia, whose background combines two great soccer traditions—growing up in Wales before returning to stardom in his native Italy, has won the scoring crown every year since he joined the Cosmos, except when he was injured in 1983. In fact, Chinaglia holds every NASL game, season, and career scoring record. One of the toughest to surpass is his having scored the winning goals in two consecutive Soccer Bowls, in 1977 and 1978. Captain of the Cosmos since 1979, Chinaglia added a unique title in 1983 when he became the owner and president of the team he had starred with in Italy between 1967 and 1976, Lazio of Rome.

Chinaglia's interest in nutrition started around the same time as his professional soccer career, when he was a sixteen-year-old apprentice with Swansea in Wales. Throughout his career, at Inter in Naples, with Lazio, and with the Cosmos, Chinaglia has tried to maintain a diet based on balance and "high quality but simple food." His breakfast is usually eggs and pancakes, followed by a light lunch based on what's fresh and available, and a dinner centered on a solid steak. He shuns desserts generally and never eats sweets.

The only variation to his menu is that three and a half hours before a game (replacing the meal usually eaten at that time) Chinaglia will have French toast and coffee. Also, in the off-season, while he follows the same basic diet he reduces the size of the portions to make up for the decrease in exercise.

The first World Cup Championship match most Americans saw was won in 1982 by the Azzurras, the Italian National Team. That game introduced two other Italian national treasures to U.S. audiences. The captain of that squad was **Dino Zoff,** who even at the age of forty is considered the premier goaltender in the world. Zoff's acclaim began when he left his native northeastern Italy to play for Naples. His greatest glories however were back north with Juventus of Turin, one of Italy's two or three most outstanding clubs, which he joined in 1971.

Zoff attributes his eating habits to three influences—his northeastern upbringing, his own observations while playing in the South, and the newspaper interviews of an English colleague. First of all, true to his regional predilections, Zoff loves meat, particularly beef and lamb, and fruit. His dislike for fish is well known throughout Italian football. He often has two slices of lamb and one of beef before matches, in addition to boiled eggs. The morning of the match against Brazil in the 1982 World Cup he was up to four slices of lamb.

Contrary to some American conceptions, pasta is not the universal basic of Italian cuisine. Generally, the farther south one goes in Italy, the more important it becomes. Zoff discovered it that way, playing in Naples. In those days it was considered inconceivable for a First Division Italian professional "footballer" to eat pasta. But Zoff, who had become a big fan of the quick thinking and imaginative Neapolitans, researched the source of their talents. The answer came from one of the local journalists who covered their games. "It's because of the carbohydrates in the pasta," he was told. That was good enough for Zoff. Unfortunately, when he went back north to Juventus, eating pasta was still considered anathema. So he used to have tons of spaghetti in the off-season, to which he attributed his fast starts early in the season.

The other main aspect of Zoff's regular diet came to him in an even more unusual way. When Arsenal, one of England's most illustrious clubs, won the Football Association Cup for the fourth time in their history in 1971, one of the stars was Bob Wilson, the goalkeeper. Zoff watched the Cup final on TV and the next day bought two or three English dailies. Thus he learned that Wilson had violated what was then the basic rule against heavy meals before day games by eating three boiled eggs on the morning of that important match. Wilson said that eggs give instant strength because the system assimilates them quickly. Again, that was enough for him. He has included them in his pregame diet ever since.

The man who was putting the ball in the back of Brazil and West Germany's nets while Zoff was barricading Italy's, was the virtually unanimous selection as the star of the 1982 World Cup

Matches, **Paolo Rossi.** Catlike reflexes, deadly acceleration, fine ball control, and excellent accuracy make him one of the most lethal forwards of all time. Also a Juventus mainstay, Rossi is fifteen years younger than his former goalkeeper, and a fellow northerner, although a Tuscan. As such, he's a staunch advocate of pasta and meat and an unwavering enemy of rice, elaborate sauces, and soft drinks.

He is also against lettuce and the like. On the other hand, artichokes (two of them were part of his pregame preparation for the startling Brazilian upset in the World Cup) and red wine, which is more fortifying than white wine, get his vote.

Zoff and Rossi may well make the All-Time World Cup team at their respective ends of the field. There is no doubt as to one entry between them, the man who revolutionized midfield play, **Franz Beckenbauer.** At Germany's two great powerhouses, Bayern Munich and Hamburg S.V., and during two stints with the Cosmos, he has won virtually every cup and award in international soccer, most notably being the captain of West Germany's World Cup Championship Team in 1978 and having the ultra-prestigious title of European Footballer of the Year both in 1972 and 1976. Back with the Cosmos, he is once again dazzling friends and foes alike with his field vision, playmaking, and deft touch.

It was when Beckenbauer was reaching his greatest heights that he first started to rethink his diet. "About ten years ago I changed my ideas about nutrition," he says. "Now I believe that a well-rounded diet, excluding junk food completely and controlling sweets is extremely important." During the season Beckenbauer will have a breakfast that consists of an English muffin, one boiled egg (even though he's not an English or an Italian goalie), and a cup of coffee. His main meal is lunch, which is built around fish and fresh vegetables. Dinner is light, just a salad with raw vegetables, cheese, and—not surprising for a man who is a native of Munich—beer. He takes a multivitamin supplement daily to round out his program.

Off-season, Beckenbauer basically maintains the same regime, but in smaller quantities. When traveling, he also follows the same schedule, except that if there is a late game he won't eat breakfast the following morning but will have a larger lunch to compensate—and much more often than not, to celebrate.

**Bob Iarusci,** a native of Toronto, is as much a rarity in soccer as a New Yorker like Nick Fotiu is in hockey. Yet Iarusci, with the Cosmos' 1982 triumph, became the first player to be in four NASL championships involving more than one team, 1976 with Toronto, 1977, 1978, and 1982 in New York, after also being the first player to be in on three consecutive championships.

Clearly a winner, Iarusci's straightforward disciplined style includes his diet. He follows just a few basic rules that include eating well-balanced meals without snacking, especially after supper. When he's home he has toast and coffee for breakfast, but will sometimes eat pancakes on a game day. Lunch is soup and a sandwich or pasta, while dinner is meat, vegetables, and a salad. When he travels he has pancakes for breakfast, a light sandwich for lunch, and a small plate of spaghetti for dinner. To end the interview I asked him if he cooked. "No," was the reply, "but I make great hero sandwiches." How appropriate!

**Glen Myernick,** who plays both defense and midfield for the Tampa Bay Rowdies, is another urban development, hailing from Trenton, New Jersey. One of America's most honored native players, Myernick won the Herman Award (soccer's Heisman) in 1976, was captain of the U.S. National Team, and a first round draft choice in the NASL.

Myernick has a very sensible attitude toward nutrition. "Sure, most of what the athletes feel about nutrition is superstitious, for example that eating a steak will give you energy. If it has before and hasn't let you down, they feel that chances are it will do it all the time for you. I take four hours to digest a steak, and some players eat it right before the game and then say it works instantly. No way. But they resist any changes. I don't want to go out on the field and worry about what I've eaten. I say I feel good because I ate right and I slept right and then I can forget about all that and concentrate on my game. If I have to think about that enormous piece of chocolate cake I ate the night before and how it will affect me, it cuts into my playing ability. If you eat well, you never have to worry about it.

"I am also a firm believer in mental toughness. Look around

and say, if other guys can do it so can I. After all, physical ability is mental as well. Examine all the aspects of your life. Question yourself. How can I change to maximize my performance? Eat, sleep, work, recreate. Don't do things just because that's what you are used to if it doesn't make sense to you now!"

For Myernick, breakfast on a training day is light, fruit, juice, and toast, or a bowl of cold cereal with milk. If he's not training that day he'll have an omelette and whole grain toast. On a game day it will be hard boiled eggs, toast, fruit, and milk at nine o'clock in the morning, and then five hours prior to the event he will have his big meal. At the team clubhouse he chooses bananas (for potassium), eggs, potatoes, spaghetti, toast, fruit juice, and ice water, and he also takes salt tablets in hot weather. Right before the game he will have more liquids, usually orange juice, water, or apple juice.

Myernick believes in a limited system of carbohydrate loading. He does it just the day before the game. Then, throughout the day, he'll have four pieces of toast, pasta, French toast or pancakes and/or his favorites, macaroni and cheese or lasagna, plus the usual protein. He follows this regime because he feels it gives him more energy for the game—not out of habit.

**Dan Canter** is a key part of the stalwart backfield unit of Team America. An All-American sweeper at Penn State, Canter is continuing the strong play he became known for around the NASL when he was a Ft. Lauderdale Striker. With Canter's help, Team America has proved it can play with anyone, especially when it comes to its tenacious defense.

Canter likes to have one good meal a day and he tries to stay away from sugar as much as possible. For breakfast he doesn't eat a lot, simply orange juice and toast. Canter generally eats lunch with the team, and it will be the biggest meal of the day. Ideally, he will have steak, spaghetti, a salad, and a bowl of soup, and he tries to eat this eight hours before the game. If he eats much later than that he feels weighed down. He is much too wound up after the game to eat dinner, so he might just have a light sandwich and a beer in the locker room. Afterward, before bed, he'll have some milk and an orange. He takes a multivitamin supplement daily and makes sure to drink a lot of fluids "as you sweat out most of your electrolytes." Off-season he has to watch the quantity of what he eats and cuts down his lunches, rather than opposing forwards.

A former teammate of Canter's and still a star with the Fort Lauderdale Strikers, **Brian Kidd** has scored many goals in his career in England and now here. He has no trouble at all in deciding on his most memorable goal. It was on his nineteenth birthday, when he was a young star for one of soccer's most illustrious teams, Manchester United. Before one hundred thousand fans in one of soccer's greatest shrines, Wembley Stadium, Kidd blasted one home in the European Cup Final.

For Kidd, eating is a way of life. His advice is to be conscious of what you're eating. "Luckily I have the advantage of not having a weight problem. Certain people have to watch themselves constantly, if they just look at a donut they'll get fat. Not me. On the other hand, I don't make a pig of myself." Diets, he feels, have to be individualized. "The athlete has to be extremely careful. If the average person wants to make a mess of his body, he generally can. Athletes, however, don't have that luxury, they are constantly being watched and their livelihood depends on it. When you're young perhaps, you can get away with it, but it eventually catches up to you."

Kidd, who is thirty-four, has been playing professionally since he was fifteen and feels that the soccer clubs in England were very helpful. They pointed out the pitfalls of being an athlete. "For example, one of their favorite sayings was 'If you want lung cancer, all you have to do is smoke.' They suggested not drinking, only a glass of wine or an occasional beer and eating the right kinds of food—fresh fruit and fish and not a lot of red meat."

Kidd has followed that advice and does not smoke or drink. Breakfast is a whole grain cereal for energy and roughage and a grapefruit, nothing fried or greasy. Lunch after practice is a poached egg and a salad. If he's tired, he'll have a protein drink consisting of milk, protein powder, and an egg yolk. He always eats whole grain bread, never white. Dinner is a salad, fish, fresh vegetables, a baked potato, plus a dessert of cheese and fruit, usually either an apple, banana, or orange.

"Remember that one man's meat is another man's poison. What's good for one is not necessarily good for someone else. On a match day my breakfast will be the same as always, and whereas for a pregame lunch the possibilities at the club are spaghetti with meat sauce, steaks, scrambled eggs, and pancakes, I opt for something lighter, just a poached egg on a slice of toast. Then right before the match I'll have some tea." Kidd does not believe in the theory of eating sweet things to boost the sugar level in his blood. "In fact, if I eat a couple of candy bars before a game I'll get sick. Energy is a long-term process which one has to work on every day." And the time to start is when you are a kid, even if you're a Kidd.

Of the twelve nationalities on the Ft. Lauderdale Strikers, the Dutch are strongly represented by one of their former Olympians, **Thomas Rongen.** Rongen is unusual in the NASL for two reasons. First, he is a foreign star who has played nearly all of his professional career to date (he's only twenty-seven) in the U.S., and he's also a highly qualified coach. Besides his teaching degree from the University of Amsterdam, Rongen has a U.S. Soccer Federation A License, the highest, as a soccer coach.

Drawing on both his playing and educational backgrounds, Rongen feels that in order to maintain the fitness needed for world class soccer, "eating well and healthfully is the perfect combination for endurance and strength. In soccer it is especially important, as you can lose up to eight pounds of fluid per game." He has found the U.S. approach to diet a big plus. "In Holland they believe that steak on the day of a game is essential. Four or five hours before a match all the players eat steak—it's traditional sports medicine. In America it's different, and I find I respond better to a more balanced diet. I do eat meat, but I've found that other proteins, such as the ones found in soybeans, are also good. In addition, vitamins are an important part of my program. A thousand milligram time-release vitamin C seems to give me more energy. I take this with a mineral supplement, a multi-vitamin capsule, ten brewer's yeast tablets (seven and a half grams per tablet), two tablespoons of raw wheat germ (toasting it destroys the vitamin E) mixed in with some plain yogurt, vitamin $B_{15}$, which I found increases endurance (one capsule a day, about ninety milligrams), and also a special product from Russia called extract from Eleutherokokkus, a form of Siberian ginseng which also improves my endurance. It comes in capsules or drops and I take thirty drops or three capsules.

"We generally practice early in the morning so my breakfast will be small. I'll have a large glass of freshly squeezed orange juice and I'll take my vitamins at that time." At noon or twelve-thirty (the games are at eight in the evening) Rongen will have a three or four ounce steak or one poached egg with either spaghetti or a baked potato, a salad, and some consommé or other clear broth. "I don't eat fruit because it is known to upset your stomach." Right before the game he might have a cup of tea with honey and a piece of toast. After the game, which usually lasts about three hours, he drinks a lot of fluids ("I generally weigh one seventy-five, but after the game I can go down to one sixty-eight") and he may have seafood, oysters, or steamers around midnight.

Rongen has taken the American path toward health food. At home, off-season, his favorite foods are salads, sprouts, nuts, almonds, sesame seeds, and fruit. His off-season breakfast is low-fat yogurt mixed with bananas, apples, oranges, and sprinkled with nuts. Lunch will be a large salad or a sandwich; one of his favorites is ham, cheese, and sprouts. Dinner is fish or chicken, with red meat once a week. "Meat gives me strength," he believes.

"The important thing is to eat small amounts of everything and to stay away from sugar and all the sweetened drinks. It is infinitely better to drink a glass of water instead of a bottle of coke, and to substitute juices (apple, orange, grape) for any soda. When you travel, as soccer players do very frequently, take something from home to eat on the plane and then just eat the vegetable and the salad that they serve you. Calcium is also important, so I drink skim milk and have a small piece of cheese every day." Staying true to his country, he likes Edam and Gouda.

"Listen to your body, it will tell you what it needs in the way of nutrition. Don't be too set in your ways. Just remember to eat a balanced diet so your body can take something from each group and have complete nutrition."

Another Dutch treat to North American soccer is **Wilhelmus "Wim" Rijsberger,** winner of the NASL's Top Defender Award in 1981. A Cosmo since 1979, Rijsberger has had two other professional homes. The first, of course, was his native Holland, where he starred both on their powerhouse Feyenoord as well as the potent national team that was a finalist in the World Cups of both 1974 and 1978. That was succeeded by a brief stop in France, actually Corsica, playing for one of their top teams, Bastia.

Through it all, Rijsberger has followed the same tight diet, only altering the schedule according to his travels. He not only avoids all junk foods, he almost avoids food altogether. Breakfast is just orange or grapefruit juice plus vitamins B complex, C, D, and E. A light lunch means dinner is the main meal—fish or chicken, fresh vegetables, and salad. At six feet and 155 pounds, Rijsberger doesn't have much margin for error in his diet.

**Rey Jaffet,** the trainer for the Fort Lauderdale Strikers, feels that the most important nutritional aspect of soccer is to drink plenty of fluids before, after, and during practice. "Water is the best. A player should have a good eight ounces of fluid every twenty minutes according to the heat of the day. When you start losing electrolytes like magnesium, calcium, and potassium you must replenish these. If not, cramps in the stomach and legs will result." Jaffet does not believe in sugared drinks and soda, as they defeat the purpose. "In order for your body to dilute the sugar," he says, "it brings the water out, so it is dehydrating you even more."

Jaffet has another bone to pick with the white stuff: "Sugar is digested in the stomach and the body turns it into fast energy. However, there is an almost immediate reaction in the pancreas to secrete insulin. As a result, a little while after eating sugar the players might become sluggish. I do not recommend sugar for an endurance sport like soccer. Some of the players have a spoonful of honey twenty minutes before the game, but some feel that after a while even this backfires and they feel more tired than before. Basically, I do not believe in quick energy for an endurance sport. I try to encourage the players to eat more complex carbohydrates which give more long-term energy. Sometimes, however, small amounts of caffeine will give a boost.

But don't drink coffee until you need it, for it won't have any effect!"

Jaffet thinks that pregame meals should be eaten at least six or seven hours before the match. As far as their content goes: "I do not recommend that players drink milk then, as it has been known to upset the stomach. Avoid roughage also and fruits that have cellulose. Salad, and heavy things like hamburgers or steak, are not ideal either, and stay away from fatty things. The object is not to have anything that will either upset the stomach or be too heavy."

Jaffet feels that protein is important to build up tissues, but that soccer players should not abuse it. "Not everyone realizes this, but protein can make you lose fluids by producing uric acid which then has to be eliminated. For this sport, I do not believe in high protein diets. If you need a great deal of protein, drink a great deal of fluids to balance it off. A balanced diet is always the best of all."

As for other soccer tips: "Be wary of refined foods, white bread, and a great deal of caffeine. Avoid too much sugar and salt. As far as salt tablets go, some players feel they will replenish what is lost in perspiration, some players need them psychologically. If that's the case, take them, but be sure to drink lots of water with them. If you take a salt tablet and it is not dissolved, it will cause bloating in the stomach, therefore, it has to be balanced with a great deal of fluids."

Jaffet is also a fan of vitamin supplements: "In Europe the players take a thousand milligrams of $B_{12}$ daily. They believe it helps their concentration, and it has been proven to help short term memory. And while there is nothing better than a balanced diet to supply the right vitamins naturally, I think a player should supplement his daily regime with a multi-vitamin, a B complex, and vitamin C."

Ken Schields, the trainer of the Tampa Bay Rowdies, feels differently about vitamins. "Americans," he says, "have the most expensive urine in the world, due to their overdosing of vitamin supplements. Unfortunately, we also have the problem of constantly being bombarded with food. Breakfast meetings, lunch meetings, dinners, etc. We don't really get a chance to let our bodies tell us what we need—and different people and nationalities have different needs. For example, our Yugoslavian player, Refik Cozic, has to eat his big meal during the day, while other players eat no lunch and need a larger dinner."

Schields does share Jaffet's views on liquids and sugars. "Fluid is important, and not the sweet stuff which takes water out of your system to balance the concentration of sugar. If you eat a lot of sugar before a game you will have a high for a few minutes and then a low. The most important energy source is carbohydrates other than sugar. Even Gatorade is a combination of potassium, sodium, chlorine, and sugar." Schields does not believe in drinking a great deal of coffee or tea before a match. He feels that while caffeine increases the metabolism of fats, if you drink too much you will lose fluids as well.

The diet of the professional soccer player is as varied as the different personalities and nationalities of the players that make up the teams. The reason many players made it to the pros has little to do with diet; a lot has to do with what they were born with. There are no special diets, foods, or food supplements that are going to make you a better athlete. However, there are a few areas concerning diet that directly affect performance on the playing field:

## The Ken Schields Primer on Soccer Nutrition

First of all, the professional must compete at a high level at all times. Both those who have reached this level of performance on God-given abilities and those who have worked their proverbial butts off to get there must maintain a high standard of physical fitness. This is where diet enters as *one of* the important factors controlling physical ability. It is almost impossible to isolate all of the elements that lead to decreasing fitness, injury, or even psychological problems. However, one factor that can be controlled and one that, when regulated properly, can show positive results is diet.

Any athlete at any level of competition should set certain standards for what he or she eats. An athlete must also remember that nutritional requirements will vary in and out of season as well as with climate.

A balanced diet (for soccer players as well as everyone else) includes proteins (the building blocks of the body), fats (a high energy

163

source), carbohydrates (the body's primary energy source), vitamins, minerals, and water. The athlete should consume about 55 to 65 percent of his or her diet in high carbohydrate foods such as breads, fruits, cakes, potatoes, vegetables, and pastries; 25 to 30 percent high fat content foods, such as butter, margarine, peanut butter, salad oils, and nuts; and 10 to 15 percent protein rich foods, such as cereals, cheese, meat, fish, liver, milk, poultry, nuts, and vegetables. Vitamins and minerals are supplied by a diet consisting of a variety of the above foods, especially vegetables.

The amount of food taken into the body can be measured in calories. An average daily caloric requirement for young men is about three thousand calories and about two thousand calories for young women. Sports activity can add as much as two or three thousand calories to the daily requirement. It takes about thirty-five hundred calories to burn off one pound of body weight. You burn up about a hundred calories for each mile you run. These figures can be helpful if you find it necessary to regulate your diet for weight loss or gain. Most products today contain a list of caloric values on their packages.

## WEIGHT GAIN OR LOSS

There are many weight loss programs available today, but there is only one successful way to lose weight. It is a combination of balanced diet, decreased daily (caloric) intake, and exercise. Losing a lot of weight in a short period of time is fairly easy; however, it can be dangerous, especially to athletes. Also, keeping quick weight loss off is very difficult.

To lose weight start by setting a realistic goal of a pound or two a week. Cut out between-meal snacks and eating anything after dinner. This may be all that is necessary. Next step is to cut down the size of your meals. If this doesn't produce sufficient loss, check the caloric values of the food that you eat most frequently. You can then cut down or eliminate the high-calorie foods. Warning! Watch what you cut out; you must keep your diet balanced. One thing you will find out quickly is that diet is more important than exercise when trying to lose weight.

Trying to gain weight is yet another problem. It seems that many of us associate bigger athletes with better athletes. This is far from being absolute. Stronger and quicker have a lot more to do with athletic performance. Gaining weight can be accomplished by a combination of a well-balanced (sound familiar?), increased-volume diet, and a program of exercise aimed at increasing strength and, if necessary, bulk. You should consult with your doctor, trainer, or coach about proper weight gaining programs.

It must also be understood that weight gain is more under the control of mother nature than yourself. Many athletes don't reach physiological growth "spurts" or maturity until they are twenty or twenty-two years old. At this point, weight gain can be easier; however, it can also become a problem. One piece of good advice—work on strength, speed, quickness, and knowledge of the game. In most cases, they are more important to your performance than extra weight.

## NUTRITIONAL SUPPLEMENTS

Most athletes can meet their nutritional requirements through balanced meals. Supplementation is rarely necessary. During hot weather, it is necessary to increase water and/or other fluid intake. Electrolyte drinks are very helpful. Taking a multiple vitamin each day is fine, but spending lots of money on extra vitamins and other nutritional supplements is not. Also, since you only need 10 to 15 percent protein in your diet, the need for protein supplements is questionable. However, if you wish to spend the money for supplements (that can't hurt you) and you feel that they help you—do it! It is your choice.

## STARTING THE DAY

Everyone should eat breakfast. It doesn't have to be a big meal, but enough to fuel the player for the morning. Experience has shown that some players will get sick during heavy morning workouts, especially if they didn't eat breakfast. They feel that a full stomach will make them ill; however, in these cases the opposite may be true, for an *empty* stomach could be the cause. The remedy is often a small breakfast, regulated by the player's particular tastes. For example, a bowl of cereal or toast, juice, and coffee or tea can be adequate.

## PREGAME NUTRITION

Good nutrition for an athlete doesn't happen on the day of the game. It is maintained all week long, every day of the year. What you eat the day of the game is very individualistic and should be controlled by what you like and digests best for you. Pregame meals should follow these guidelines:

1. Don't eat too close to game time. Your system should be concentrating on your muscles and brain during the game, not on your digestive system. Three to four hours or longer before starting time is recommended.
2. Don't eat a lot of hard-to-digest foods such as protein (meats) and fats.
3. Eat mostly carbohydrates (pasta, pancakes, toast, etc.). They are easy to digest and a good energy source.
4. Don't eat spicy foods. If you like pastas such as spaghetti, be sure to have them with a mild, unseasoned, or slightly seasoned sauce.
5. Don't eat gas-producing foods. You must know which foods affect you in this way. Stay clear of them.
6. This is a good time to start building up your fluids. Orange juice is good for this. Too much coffee and tea can have the opposite effect, as can any drink with caffeine.

When trying to plan meals it is most practical to select foods that are (a) easy to prepare, (b) readily available, and (c) nutritionally sound.

In order to help you plan your daily diets, here is an example of a daily diet plan:

*Breakfast*    fruit juice
cereal with milk or skim milk and fruit
(optional)
toast (whole wheat), butter and jelly
coffee, tea, or milk

*Lunch*    soup and/or salad
sandwich (on whole wheat or rye)
milk, soft drink, or fruit juice
fresh fruit for dessert

*Dinner*
soup and/or salad
rolls and butter or margarine
fish, poultry, or meat (in that order), broiled or baked
water, milk, or soft drink
coffee or tea and dessert of choice

## Guidelines

1. Take it easy on coffee and tea. Too much caffeine is not good for soccer players.
2. Eat to satisfy your hunger, not until you're *full.*
3. During the preseason especially, or in season, when you are fatigued, you may lose your appetite. This is when you must be careful to maintain an adequate intake of both food and liquids.
4. Drink plenty of fluids, especially before games or practice even if you are not thirsty. If it makes you uncomfortable, drink less, but you must "hydrate" yourself before you start! Drink water with every meal.
5. If your practice sessions or games are in the afternoon, eat a bigger breakfast (for example, add eggs and bacon, or pancakes or waffles to the morning meal). Have a smaller lunch (for example, eliminate salad, have a small sandwich) and the same size dinner—but not directly after your activity—wait at least an hour or more.
6. If you practice or play at night, eat a larger breakfast, a bigger lunch (or substitute your dinner for lunch), and have only a snack after your activity.
7. Snacks should best consist of fruits, nuts, and occasionally vegetables (example, carrots and celery sticks).
8. Don't abuse your intake of alcoholic beverages. (Drinking alcoholic beverages leads to fluid loss).
9. Point to ponder: It takes a great deal of discipline to be a good soccer player. Why not use some of that discipline to be a good eater!

# CHAPTER EIGHT

# Tennis

A sprint lasts seconds. Somewhat longer races on land and water, plus the occasional boxing match, might take less than a minute or two, while most team sport events go for around an hour of game time and usually two to three hours total. Even golf tournaments last only four days. The major tennis tournaments, however, generally require at least two weeks of matches (often singles, doubles, and mixed doubles) that can easily go on for hours, especially on the slower surfaces like clay. Besides stamina, great reflexes and hand-to-eye coordination, upper body strength, extraordinary foot speed, and overall flexibility are the hallmarks of the big guns in both women's and men's tennis. It is no surprise then that world class tennis players have to be as fit as any athlete in any sport.

Tennis stars have other problems, though, besides the grueling matches. First of all, their schedules are uniquely irregularly timed. The start of the match may vary during a single event from morning to nighttime. And depending upon if and when they lose, they may either have no chance at all to prepare for the next tournament (and frequently travel to the next country across several time zones) or they may have more than a week. Equally hard on conditioning, although much more welcome to many players—at least at first—is the attention of the glitterati and associated deluxe partying that big-time tennis and its huge purses have seemed to attract. It is awfully difficult to keep on a regimented diet with room service at the Hotel George V and canapés at Régine's at your beck and call.

Nevertheless, the great players who manage to succeed for longer than one brief shining moment know that concentration and discipline (although not necessarily good manners) are the only way to stay on top. Plus, of course, the right diet. This chapter is devoted, ladies first, to the nutritional regimes of the stars of the game, advice of their coaches, and a special section and diet by former World Championship Tennis trainer Steve Parker.

**Chris Evert Lloyd** has won more Grand Slam singles titles than any other woman in today's tennis, including four straight U.S. Open Championships between 1975 and 1978. Almost unbeatable on the clay surfaces she was raised playing on in Florida, Evert Lloyd has been ranked in the top three in the world virtually continuously for nearly ten years.

For Evert Lloyd, the most important meal is the one she eats the night before a match. She'll have a steak, salad, and vegetables plus fruit for dessert. She'll also have a carbohydrate such as spaghetti to give her more energy for the match the next day. Breakfast on the game day will be light, a glass of fresh orange juice plus a boiled egg on toast and bacon. If Evert Lloyd has no match that day, she'll also have a cup of coffee. With breakfast she takes a multiple vitamin, an iron tablet, and extra vitamin C. Lunch will be a sandwich, generally turkey with cheese and mustard, and a large glass of skim milk. Evert Lloyd likes fish and chicken for dinner as well as red meat, but the other thing she loves, desserts, have been drastically cut back. "I have stopped eating chocolate, donuts, and most sweets, and because of this I have lost seventeen pounds bringing my weight from one hundred thirty-five down to one eighteen."

"Eating well is part of our profession," she says. "Sugar gives you energy for ten to fifteen minutes but then you experience an enormous drop. It is better to keep your energy up with proteins and especially with carbohydrates.

"I was also drinking about six cans of diet soda a day and I found that it was more difficult for me to lose weight even though I was not eating all that much. The diet sodas have salt in them and this retains water. When I cut them out, I lost weight as well. Now I just drink water, six to eight glasses a day. It is also a wonderful appetite suppressor."

For those who think that all the energy Evert Lloyd expends on the court is natural, it's really an effort. "I'm normally not a hyper person so I have to push myself every day." What gives her the drive, however, is sleep. "I must get at least nine hours every night. That means in bed before midnight and sleeping until nine the next morning." So much for deluxe parties.

The all-time money-earning champion with over five million dollars in prizes, **Martina Navratilova** has dominated the game throughout the long season in an unprecedented way. Combining unusual power, gymnastic flexibility, and great speed, Navratilova at the top of her game is almost unbeatable. Just ask Andrea Jaeger who lost to Navratilova in the 1983 Wimbledon Finals in the astonishingly short time of fifty-four minutes.

As a Czech emigré, Navratilova had a lot of adjustments to make in coming to America, including diet. After a great deal of searching and many problems, she has finally settled down to a special diet that was devised for her by her nutritionist, Dr. Robert Haas. "Martina is the first Bionic Athlete," says Haas, who feels that eating the right diet can improve endurance and performance, prevent injury, and extend career longevity—as it does for Navratilova. In designing her diet, Haas took into account her blood pressure, body weight, body fat, number of calories required during exercise, and her individual tastes. He then feeds all this into a computer and the results will be what she needs to obtain peak performance.

There are a few basic rules to Haas's diet. He believes that the ideal program should be extremely low in fat, high in such complex carbohydrates as potatoes, spaghetti, and bread (without butter or cheese toppings), fresh fruit, and unlimited vegetables. He believes that the biggest health offenders are, in increasing order, cholesterol, excess fats, excess proteins, salt, and sugar.

Although Navratilova is addicted to fruit, especially peaches, tangerines, oranges, and apples, she does have a sweet tooth, which has to be taken into consideration. Haas has even come up with a special (and unfortunately secret) recipe for chocolate cake.

Her basic rules are no red meat, no oils, and a very high intake of carbohydrates like pasta, spaghetti, and potatoes. She will also have broiled chicken and fish, steamed vegetables, and mixed salad. When in training, a typical day for Navratilova would be buckwheat pancakes for breakfast, tuna on whole wheat for lunch followed by an apple, a slice of melon, and a banana. Dinner would be spaghetti, salad, and fresh fruit for dessert.

Says Haas: "I change Martina's diet based on whether she's playing a tournament or training. For example I'll tell her 'This week you have to have at least five ounces of low-fat animal protein daily'; another day she might substitute beans for animal protein, or she might concentrate on fish." Better playing through chemistry.

The mantle of *grande dame* of lady's tennis rests uneasily on **Billie Jean King**'s shoulders. With an incredible twenty Wimbledon titles (six in singles) to go with her French, Australian, and four U.S. Open wins, King is still playing and winning in competition with kids who weren't even born when she was taking her first titles.

It was back in the early 1970's that King changed her ideas on nutrition. She discovered that many of the things in her diet were making her tired and she was not playing up to her peak performance. Having learned from this experience, her advice for players interested in tennis is: "Eat right now. Learn about fitness young and you'll have a better life. Also don't start drinking alcohol; it can really hinder your performance."

Other *don'ts* for King include candy, dairy products, caffeine in all forms, sugar, diet sodas, or any kind of junk food. Her *do's* are simple—just a good balanced diet augmented by vitamin and mineral supplements including vitamins A, B complex, C, and D along with zinc, selenium, iron, and calcium.

A sensation as a teenager with her then innovative two-handed style, **Tracy Austin** has gone on to prove her potential already, having two U.S. Open Singles Titles to her credit. At five feet, four inches and a slender 110 pounds, Austin must constantly watch her weight. To keep trim, she chooses meals of salads, light animal proteins such as chicken or fish, and lots of fruit and vegetables. Like King, she eats no fats, sweets, or dairy products, and drinks plenty of water. That leaves her just twenty Wimbledon titles behind.

**Carling Bassett,** number-one women's player in Canada, is the first Canadian woman to do well in the major international circuit and was the second youngest on tour in 1983. She caught the public's fancy in the Amelia Islands WTA Championship Match, where she forced Chris Evert Lloyd to three sets—a rarity on Evert Lloyd's home Florida clay. Tennis's newest sensation, she has a very definite idea of nutrition. Because she is only in her mid-teens, however, she can afford to eat things that the older players try to avoid, french fries, for example, and one of her favorite dishes—pan pizza.

In general, though, Bassett's teenage diet is as exceptional as her teenage tennis talents. If she is playing a late morning match she will have a large breakfast. This consists of a boiled egg, a glass of juice (always freshly squeezed) plus a piece of whole grain toast with honey. She will also have a bowl of Grape Nuts for more carbohydrates and on a match day she uses salt since she loses so much of it on the court.

After the match, Bassett will head toward the salad bar and have a sandwich along with it, her favorites being egg salad, tuna fish, or roast beef. If Bassett is playing at night, she will only eat a baked potato or french fries, with ice cream for dessert. "My favorite snacks are raw vegetables, celery, broccoli, and carrots, which I have with a blue cheese dip.

"I'm really not a big eater as I don't like the feeling of a heavy stomach, nor do I drink sugar drinks. I realize that I can get away with eating more now, but I'll have to cut down when I reach nineteen." It's always good to plan for your old age.

**Sylvia Hanika** is another young national number one, being the top woman tennis player of West Germany. Besides her lofty international ranking, Hanika is one of the few women who can boast of conquests over Navratilova. Although a Munich native, Hanika belies her German upbringing by adhering to a more or less American way of nutrition.

For breakfast, Hanika has cereal with scrambled eggs followed by some low-fat yogurt for calcium. Lunch is a large green salad that she seeks out everywhere, even on tour. On this she puts an oil and vinegar dressing and will have it with a few slices of whole grain toast. She has found that this is all she needs to get her through an afternoon of playing—along with the only liquid she drinks, water. Dinner is her largest meal of the day. Steak ("I love filet mignon"), fish, or chicken are the key elements. Carbohydrates come from either her German standby, noodles, or spaghetti. "Vitamins are also important and I use a multi-vitamin powder which I sprinkle on my food. I find this easier to take and to digest." Hanika likes ice cream which she will occasionally indulge in, but her favorite foods of all are Bavarian, cooked by her mother. Unfortunately for Hanika, though, bratwurst and break points don't go well together.

**Lisa Bonder** is a youngster in the top twenty-five and an example of an eighteen-year-old who started early learning about nutrition. "I used to be a junk food addict," she says, "but I find I have more energy if I eat properly." Bonder does not have a weight problem and feels that the more you exercise, the more you should eat.

For breakfast, Bonder will have three or four waffles with syrup plus bacon on the side. "The waffles are a high energy carbohydrate and the bacon adds protein." Additional vitamins come from a multiple supplement plus C and E. Lunch is not an important meal for her, so she usually just has some fruit, such as a banana for potassium and an orange. Or else she'll have salad with some cottage cheese on top. During the day, she gets fluids and energy from grapefruit and orange juice. Dinner is always heavy in carbohydrates. "I don't eat too much red meat but I do eat a lot of fish and chicken and have this with spaghetti or pasta. Another dish that is not so bad for you is pizza; it has cheese for protein, bread for carbohydrates, and tomato sauce, high in vitamin C. If it is made well it is a high-energy food. Another wonderful dinner is soft shell tacos. I take some enchilada shells, the soft kind, and fill them with chicken, a slice of tomato, sharp cheddar cheese and put a little butter and lettuce in them, and then just roll them up and eat them." Bonder's

173

advice for traveling: "No matter where you are, look for a salad bar and you can always have a good fresh meal."

**Janice Alvord** is the masseuse for the Women's Tennis Association. The WTA, which was founded in 1973 at King's inspiration, has named among its presidents the great stars, including most recently Navratilova. Alvord travels the WTA circuit and attends to the players right before they go out on the court. She is the equivalent of the trainer in other sports. Alvord feels that massage therapy, while it won't cause you to lose or gain weight, is an important adjunct to proper diet. "Regular massages," she contends, "help reduce injury and illness by cleaning out the lymphatic system. Europeans believe in the power of massage to break down the lactic acid and put it back into the bloodstream to be eliminated. It also lowers stress and tension. All tennis players should have massages routinely. Don't wait until you are sore!"

As far as nutrition goes, Alvord has some tips there as well: "Drink plenty of liquids; eat a normal, healthy, well-rounded diet with everything in moderation and nothing in excess. Remember that as you get older your metabolism slows down so you have to cut down on your calorie intake and exercise twice as much to keep in shape. Stay away from fats and cholesterol if you want to avoid cellulite, those lumpy 'orange rind' deposits that women get on their hips and thighs. The midriff, hips, and thighs and underneath the bicep area is where most women have problems and it is only through exercise and a balanced diet that you can achieve good results and keep these firm and slim. In combination it will make you a better tennis player." Alvord's advice for dealing with international time change is basic common sense: "Take a few days off when you first arrive wherever you're going to get your inner time clock back in order." Unless you've got a match the next day.

On the men's side, the matches tend to be considerably longer (playing best three out of five in major tournaments, versus two out of three for the women) and therefore the conditioning is even more critical. While, as in all sports, the desire and mental toughness have to be there, so does the fuel to keep the motor running.

**Ivan Lendl** has won everything in sight except a Grand Slam title. In 1982, he broke the prize money record by winning over two million dollars. He also set a record for matches won, 106 out of 115, while taking fifteen out of twenty-three tournaments. His victories include the 1981 and 1982 Volvo Masters, the 1982 WCT Finals and the Association of Tennis Professionals Championships in 1982. Always among the world's top three players, Lendl is a product of the same great Czechoslovakian national tennis program that bred Navratilova.

Lendl is very much a believer that nutrition is important in the life of an athlete. And while he takes no vitamins, he has throughout his life made an effort to eat healthfully.

Lendl's diet concentrates on high quality proteins which he feels gives him more energy. If his match schedule allows, his first meal will usually be around ten-thirty in the morning and will consist of eggs, bacon, bread, and orange juice or lemonade. Lunch, if he's playing a late afternoon match, will then be a club or steak sandwich, and dinner will once again concentrate on meat, either steak or something lighter, such as veal or chicken, and always hot soup. When he plays he eats a great deal of the above—shades of Wayne Gretzky—while between tournaments the menu remains about the same but the portions will be smaller.

The bottom line for Lendl is to avoid any kind of food that will upset his stomach. To that end he eats only plain foods and has his main courses broiled and his vegetables steamed. A very sensible diet befitting a very sensible person. And to make sure he can get his meals this way (although there are possibly other reasons too), Lendl has mastered eight languages along with hitting tennis balls. His favorite foods, however, are those cooked by his mother, and they are, of course, in Czech.

A man of many titles and talents, **John Newcombe,** winner of the Singles Title at Wimbledon in 1967, 1970, and 1971, the U.S. Open in 1967 and 1973, the Australian Open in 1973 and 1975, and the WCT Finals in 1974, is now a successful sports journalist, commercial actor, and, according to John, "the best short order cook in the world. You name it, I'll do it." What he won't do, however, is eat "rubbish," presumably the Aussie equivalent of junk food. His advice for younger players is to stay away from junk food and learn to know what your body best responds to by practical experience.

As a man whose prime athletic career spanned the time when more attention among both health and sports professionals was given to diet, Newcombe changed his ideas about nutrition along the way as well. Like Lendl, his diet evolved into one based on first-class animal protein—steak, fish, liver, and chicken, even eggs and bacon "when I feel like it." However, before a match a large dose of complex carbohydrate food is added, his favorites being baked beans, which he has along with vegetables and fruit. When he's not playing, to keep his weight down, he simply cuts back on the carbohydrates and continues to eat protein. Newcombe rounds off his program with supplements that include B complex, C, and E vitamins plus calcium and magnesium.

Almost at the other end of the dietary spectrum from Lendl and Newcombe is another one of Dr. Haas's patients, **Gene Mayer,** who credits better diet with contributing to his improved standing to the top five worldwide. Mayer, who was a mainstay of the U.S. Davis Cup win in 1982, never really ate junk food, but his diet had been high in fats and sugars and too much animal protein. "I realized how poorly I had felt compared to my new found stamina, endurance, and high-level energy. I now need less sleep, eight hours as opposed to nine, and I feel much better in general. Not only tennis but my running has improved."

Mayer's diet is well balanced, but with a marked cant away from red meat. For breakfast he will have a cold cereal like Grape Nuts with skim milk and fruit, usually including sliced bananas. Occasionally he has pancakes. Lunch is all types of salads, generally based on a mixture of lettuce, cabbage, and beets, with chickpeas or the occasional portion of tuna fish for protein. "A wonderful dressing is vinegar with a sprinkling of Parmesan cheese over the salad. Sometimes I'll have cole slaw with a dressing of yogurt instead of mayonnaise."

Dinner is now much less meat and more substitutions, like lima beans or dried white beans warmed with garlic. Sometimes it will be pasta and a four-ounce serving of chicken, turkey, or fish. "Potatoes are also good. Dessert is always fruit and some-times a frozen yogurt. I snack on carrots, celery, and pretzels, and find that drinking orange juice mixed with seltzer is better than any soda.

"Also now with everyone making pasta it is possible to find carrot, spinach, and artichoke flours, and instead of the pack-aged breads try to find fresh whole grain ones. I now find myself looking for bread and pasta shops where before I looked for good butchers." He should give Lendl and Newcombe his old address book.

**Pancho Segura,** from one of tennis's lesser known hotbeds, Ecuador, was a champion in the 1950's and for ten years one of the top players in the world. Best known for inventing the two-handed backhand, Segura now is the tennis pro at the exclu-sive La Costa Spa and Country Club outside San Diego. Here players and would-be professionals come from the world over to take lessons from him. Not only does he comment on the tennis serve, but he feels that what is served at the table is equally important. The diet that he follows himself is the basic healthy one he recommends for everyone. Some of his students have done fairly well with it, including a fellow whom Segura coached intensely for years—a kid by the name of Jimmy Con-nors.

Some of Segura's basic rules: "First and foremost avoid all junk food, that means white bread, pastries, ice creams, cakes, and cookies. Too much fat and fried foods are not good either. Substitute plain broiled for all fried foods and make sure that all pastries are whole grain products (like bran and corn muffins). Avoid white sugar as well, and never drink soft drinks. Substi-tute plain water for sodas whenever possible."

Breakfast should be a balanced meal. "I have eggs twice a week, boiled or poached, plus a slice of whole grain toast. On the other days I'll have cereal. (Read the ingredients and look out for salt and sugar on the label. Have the pure kind.)" Or he might have a plain yogurt with bananas, papaya, and a spoonful of honey on top. Segura has a freshly squeezed glass of grapefruit juice daily, and recommends fresh juices for a quick energy pickup, though his ideal pregame drink is tea with honey.

"Lunch is a sandwich on whole grain bread, either tuna fish

| MEAL | Monday | Tuesday | Wednesday | Thursday | Friday | Saturday |
|---|---|---|---|---|---|---|
| **Breakfast** | scrambled eggs sausage patties biscuits Tater Tots cereal-toast fruit | French toast waffles bagels danish cereal-toast fruit | pancakes sausage links cereal-toast fruit | bagels French toast waffles donuts cereal-toast fruit | scrambled eggs sausage biscuits Tater Tots cereal-toast fruit | French toast waffles bagels danish cereal-toast fruit |
| **Lunch** | assorted sandwiches salad fruit | beef and shrimp chop suey steamed rice, Oriental vegetables tossed salad fruit | assorted sandwiches chicken & rice soup salad fruit | beef tacos w/lettuce, cheese and tomato garnish corn tossed salad | assorted sandwiches salad fruit | hot dogs baked beans potato chips fruit salad |

| MEAL | Monday | Tuesday | Wednesday | Thursday | Friday | Saturday |
|------|--------|---------|-----------|----------|--------|----------|
| Dinner | baked Salisbury steaks and beef stew oven-browned potatoes peas and carrots tossed salad | char-broiled steaks baked potato vegetable tossed salad | baked chicken yellow rice mixed vegetables tossed salad | Italian-style spaghetti with meat sauce broccoli salad | fried fish clam strips mackerel french fries corn/salad | veal cutlets with gravy mashed potatoes vegetable fruit salad |

| MEAL | Monday | Tuesday | Wednesday | Thursday | Friday | Saturday |
|---|---|---|---|---|---|---|
| **Breakfast** | scrambled eggs biscuits Tater Tots sausage patties cereal-toast fruit | French toast waffles bagels danish cereal-toast fruit | pancakes sausage links cereal-toast fruit | French toast waffles bagels donuts cereal-toast fruit | scrambled eggs sausage patties biscuits Tater Tots cereal-toast fruit | French toast waffles bagels danish cereal-toast fruit |
| **Lunch** | assorted sandwiches salad/fruit potato chips | ravioli carrots tossed salad fruit | assorted sandwiches soup tossed salad fruit | grilled ham and cheese baked beans tossed salad fruit | and assorted sandwiches | chicken cutlet sandwich on a bun cole slaw fruit salad |
| **Dinner** | Salisbury steaks with white rice mixed vegetables salad | roast beef red potatoes green beans tossed salad | spaghetti peas garlic bread salad | chicken rice carrots tossed salad | custom-cut cod/clam strips french fries tossed salad corn | pork chops oven-browned potatoes |

or cheese (cheddar or Swiss, never the processed American type) along with a small salad. Or just a fresh fruit salad which is full of vitamins and minerals." Dinner will start with a salad (with a dressing of safflower oil and vinegar) plus fish, twice a week, meat once a week (including liver, "very important for iron") and chicken or veal the rest of the time. The occasional glass of wine is okay, but that's it. Segura also recommends baked potatoes and his favorite vegetables are string beans and cauliflower. "The best thing to ask for in a restaurant is anything plain broiled plus a salad and a vegetable. You will never go wrong!"

Segura's playing and coaching are both long-running success stories. The newest name at the top of tennis training now is the **Nick Bolletteri's Tennis Academy,** brought to you by the same people who own the New York Cosmos—Warner Communications. The Nick Bolletteri Tennis Academy specializes in training the young stars of the circuit. Chip Hooper, Pablo Arroya, Brian Gottfried, and Pam Casale along with Bonder and Bassett have all come to brush up on their strokes. Here is what young champions eat at this tennis prep school to maximize their energy. Remember, though, these diets are intended for active teenagers.

The most dominant player in men's tennis today has to be **John McEnroe,** whose victories are legion—notably Wimbledon in 1981 and 1983, the U.S. Open in 1979, 1980, and 1981 and the Davis Cup in 1978, 1979, 1981, and 1982; besides being part of the number one doubles team in the world. There are many reasons for his success, most of which he's keeping secret. Here's one that got away, though, his favorite dish—his mother's lasagna.

## LASAGNA

Ingredients:
2–3 tbsps. olive oil
1 clove garlic
1 small chopped onion

1 lb. chopped meat
2 lb. 12 oz. can of *plum* tomatoes
½ lb. Italian sausages
1 6 oz. can tomato paste
1 lb. box of lasagna noodles
2 lbs. ricotta
2 or 3 eggs
parsley
salt and pepper
Parmesan cheese (good cheese—a poor cheese can ruin it)
1 lb. mozzarella

Brown garlic and onion lightly in olive oil. Remove garlic and onion and reserve. Brown chopped meat well. Do not let water collect.

Mash tomatoes well. Return onion and garlic to saucepot with chopped meat and add sausages. Add tomatoes, cover and simmer for two hours. *Add no water.*

Add paste to sauce. Stir occasionally. Cook over low heat for one hour. Leave uncovered. Add water when necessary. Remove sausages when through.

Cook noodles according to directions. In large bowl mix ricotta, eggs, two tbsps. snipped parsley; salt and pepper to taste. Add a good handful of Parmesan cheese (about ¼ cup).

In 14" × 10" × 2" pan, spread a quarter of sauce. Lay a third of the lasagna noodles one at a time in pan until bottom is entirely covered. Spread half of ricotta over noodles, top with a third of the mozzarella, cut in thin slices. Repeat the layers. Sprinkle top layer of noodles with some more grated Parmesan cheese, spread with remaining sauce, and top with remaining slices of mozzarella. (This can be prepared early in the day and refrigerated until ready to cook.)

Bake one hour in 400° oven. Let it stand for fifteen to thirty minutes so it will cut easily. Heat any remaining sauce for those who wish it. Heat sausages in sauce.

A trainer's view of the sports world is unique, the inside but neither a performer nor a coach. Steve Parker has had a chance to observe both the tennis and soccer scenes from that vantage. The following are some of his thoughts and remembrances about the diet and lifestyle of his world-class athletes:

## Steve Parker's Journal

My career as an athletic trainer has taken me to forty-odd countries over an eight-year period. I have just finished a year and a half with World Championship Tennis working with the best tennis players in the world. Before that I was in professional soccer, traveling nationally and internationally with the National, Junior National, and Olympic teams.

I've counseled players on diets as well as ordering food for a team over a three-month tour. With the soccer players I've found that their appetites usually adapt to their high-energy output. If a player needs to gain or lose weight then we would add or subtract calories as needed. I've found that the younger players have a tendency to live on junk food. Hamburgers were the staple with or without secret sauce and cheese. They would skip breakfast and then wonder why they were so tired after practice. With the young single player, I tried to push them toward a cafeteria and started them on a good multi-vitamin supplement. I believe in the basic balanced meal with a loading of carbohydrates the night before and day of a game.

I try to be flexible in my suggestions due to the problem of getting the required food in a foreign country. With the soccer schedule you can usually control the food intake on an extended road trip or tour. With tennis players, the schedule changes from day to day and any consistencies in time of food intake change with it. They usually eat when they are hungry, which may or may not agree with habits of good diet. The food available is also a problem. You could be in a town that shuts down at 10:00 P.M. After a late-night match, you find yourself tired and hungry with only room service of cold sandwiches and hors d'oeuvres. Because of these odd eating hours, the body's natural time clock is out of sync with your eating schedule. Diarrhea and constipation are common problems. Egg rolls and shrimp cocktails at 2:00 A.M. are no substitute for a well-balanced meal. This is why I stress the taking of a multi-vitamin at all times.

When traveling, you can run up against some unusual problems in setting up diets. We were on a tour which took us from Australia to Hong Kong and Red China. Not being a fan of Oriental food, I was dreading the trip to the Far East. The hotel in Australia where we would eat all our meals only had a Chinese restaurant. My nightmares were answered—two weeks of Chinese food before we even set foot on the Mainland.

In Shanghai we had an evening with the local dignitaries. The meal consisted of a turntable of appetizers with five courses of assorted green, red, gray, and brown unidentifiable masses on plates and in bowls. Drinks consisted of wine with a grain alcohol chaser. When the turntable of surprises hit us, presumably being the most expendable member of the group, I was appointed official food tester for our table. There were over twenty dishes and I couldn't figure out what anything was. I did all right until I got to the little brownish-red balls. The minute one touched my tongue I knew there was no way it was going any farther toward my stomach. We are talking *hot.* I immediately pushed it to the side of my mouth and left it there until I could find a polite way to roll it out again. By the time I got it out of my mouth a red welt had formed on the outside of my cheek. On to Peking!

At a state dinner in the Great Hall of the People, they had a buffet laid out. There were two entrees I tried to steer my players away from. One was a dish that resembled a rubber tube cut in half with slime added for flavor. While I found out it was intestines, I was afraid to ask whose or what's. The other dish was what is affectionately known as thousand-year-old eggs. They take eggs and bury them in the ground for ten years and dig them up and dive in. Ten years in the ground does wonders for eggs. The yellows turn black and the whites turn an opaqued gray. This is all petrified together as if someone had boiled it first.

On my first U.S. Soccer National Team trip in 1976, I developed a great weight-loss diet. In two weeks you can lose fifteen pounds. You must first find a way to get two consecutive sleepless nights on an airplane. The second night will be a late-nighter to Bogotá, Colombia. You will arrive at 4:00 A.M. to be greeted by local officials who insist you go out drinking. You finally get to bed at 7:00 A.M. and at 8:00 you are in the bathroom for your first of many episodes to follow. After one week the diet has progressed far enough to bring on hallucinations. In Quito, Ecuador at 2:00 A.M. a doctor is called in to stop your babbling so your roommate can sleep. It is important not to get a good doctor, and preferably one who speaks no English. Look for one, like mine, who does veterinarian work on the side. Now this visit from the doctor won't help your "diet" any, but I guarantee you will not ask for a doctor again. After another week in Peru and Venezuela the diet is complete and you've lost at least fifteen pounds.

In professional tennis the diets were much more varied than soccer. The players came from all over the world bringing with them the habits of their individual countries. My soccer traveling experiences did in fact pay off in that I was more apt to cope with the cuisines of different countries where the tournaments were held. The players themselves were more or less able to survive, if not thrive, by changing their eating habits to fit what was on the plate in front of them. Each country had its own specialty and I tried to fit that local flavor in any recommendations I made. The best country for a tennis pro's diet is Italy. The different ways they fix pasta made a high complete carbohydrate diet varied and tasty. The only problem I have with Italy, as well as the rest of Europe, is their salads. Roughage is essential for regularity as well as cleaning out our gastrointestinal system. Europe has a limited amount of salads on their menus and their dressings, as far as I am concerned, are usually simple and mundane. Of course, the countries to be avoided by the touring pros are the underdeveloped ones. Due to economic conditions the food is usually limited in variety and quality. Because of these problems, fats and heavy spices are used to add different tastes and textures to the food. Both these additives can play havoc with our lower tract as well as slowing the absorption time of the food we are trying to digest. My biggest complaint about these countries, though, is the high bacteria level in the food. Because of the lack of proper refrigeration, food is often left out in the elements which speeds decaying and rapid bacteria growth. Food not picked, purchased, and eaten the same day should be subject to scientific analysis before being eaten. Another big problem in underdeveloped countries is an adequate water supply. Water is usually undrinkable by anyone but the native population due to the bacteria levels. Unfortunately, this same water is used to wash and prepare much of the food eaten.

Some of the players' eating habits just couldn't adapt to the local cuisine and restaurants featuring their native specialties were sought out to satisfy their culinary cravings. The most notorious player on the circuit for seeking out his homeland's food is Vijay Amitraj. No matter where the tournament was, he always found the nearest Indian restaurant to get a plate of curry, usually on the advice of local Indian fans.

Guillermo Vilas adapted his native specialty into a weight loss diet. Argentina is known for its succulent beef and Vilas went on a meat and water diet. He ate all the meat he wanted while drinking a gallon and a half of water daily. Put this together with his four to six hours of workouts each day and he was taking off three to five pounds a week. The problem with this diet is that you can't stay on it for long and once you go back to your normal routine the weight comes right back. Fortunately for Vilas, the tennis pro has very little routine in his life and cutting down on calories is as easy as forgetting to eat a meal. The healthiest way to lose weight is to establish how many calories it takes for you to maintain your current weight. Then you cut out three to five thousand calories a week to get a slow, steady weight loss. A well-balanced diet should be maintained and if you increase your exercise load then you won't have to cut as many calories out of your diet.

Probably the most improved diet on the circuit belongs to McEnroe. At the 1982 Dallas World Championship Tennis Finals, he came into the locker room eating fried tortilla chips. It seems these were his breakfast and lunch. That night he got into a five-set battle with Bill Scanlon. After the match he was totally exhausted. His body had run out of fuel. A year later at Forest Hills I questioned McEnroe about what he had eaten for his pregame meal. A well balanced, high caloric breakfast was the answer, which proved to me that his ever striving to improve his game is extending well beyond his practice time on the court.

I've found that tennis players, due to their lifestyle, are more disciplined than the average person. Most tennis pros travel the circuit alone. It takes a tremendous amount of discipline to practice every day and even more sticking to a diet. It's so much easier to just eat the food that's available. Most of the time you really have to work at a diet while on tour. I know from my own experience with the long tournament hours that it is impossible to have good eating habits.

It seemed to go hand in hand, that as a player rose in the ranking and made more and more money his eating habits changed. If ranked over two hundred, a player is more or less struggling to make a living on the circuit. His diet may consist of hamburgers and french fries for lunch and dinner after skipping breakfast. As the players begin to do better on the court, the nicer restaurants with their richer foods are visited quite often. Then, once up to the top five in the world, if a player stays on the top long enough for his face to be very familiar to the public, going out to eat becomes a big headache. At this stage the player is limited to the local hotel room-service menu—which in some places means hamburgers and french fries.

At our Hilton Head tournament we had only night matches. It was around 11:00 P.M. and a few of the players were hanging out in the players' lounge. I was hungry and was going to order room service. Lendl said he hadn't eaten either and called room service. I told Lendl I wanted a light meal and he ordered for both of us. When the food arrived, the bill was close to a hundred dollars. There was enough food for five people. Lendl ate about a third of it and the rest was eaten by the remaining players and me. Lendl had just finished a three-hour match so the caloric intake was about right for him, but this is a good example of eating when you have a chance on the circuit.

Finally, I remind the players that, as in most professional sports, there is a problem with retirement. Your eating habits have adapted to a high-energy requirement. When a player becomes inactive, he must cut down on his caloric intake or apply for a job as the Goodyear blimp. Fortunately for most tennis pros, their retirement, if they actually do retire and not join the Senior Masters Tour, is an active one of coaching or teaching.

The following is a diet which I try to recommend to the pros that come to me for help. Breakfast is the most important meal of the day. You have slept for six to ten hours and your body has run out of fuel.

> *Breakfast:*  fruit or fruit juice
> portion of meat
> eggs twice a week
> cereal (cold or hot)
> toast, pancakes, or sweet rolls
> plus multi-vitamin supplement

Many people can't eat a big breakfast in the morning so for these people lunch should be the biggest meal of the day. Why lunch and not dinner? Because what you eat for lunch is pretty much burned up by the time you go to sleep. What you eat for dinner is digested during sleep. Due to the low energy requirement of sleeping, the calories not burned during the night are stored as glycogen and fats. The glycogen will be burned the next morning at practice but the fats will more than likely be stored away until caloric intake is cut down in the future. In addition, if dinner is late it will interfere with getting a good night's sleep.

> *Lunch:*  salad
> soup
> portion of meat or fish
> one or more green vegetables
> one other green vegetable, noodles, or bread
> milk, fruit juice, or water
> dessert—fruit

Lunch should be eaten as your energy source for the afternoon and evening. Dinner should be eaten only to keep you from going to bed hungry. If you have a match to play the next day then a larger high carbohydrate meal is in order.

*Dinner:* chef's salad
or
soup and sandwich
or
fruit salad

The size of the portions are all related to your caloric needs and whether you want to gain, lose, or maintain your weight.

# CHAPTER NINE

# Swimming

Anyone who has ever attempted the breaststroke, not to mention something really impossible like the butterfly, knows that advanced drowning is easier to master. Yet the lure of the water is so strong that fine young athletes the world over spend hours every day trying to do things that evolution left behind eons ago, turning themselves into creatures suited only for prune ads.

Competitive swimming is also a sport in which Americans have traditionally excelled. The Olympics were our private hunting grounds until the East Germans started building better (well, at least stronger) female bodies through chemistry. Nevertheless, the U.S. Men's and Women's Swimming and Diving Teams remain world powerhouses and our coaching has attracted talented athletes from around the world to our colleges.

And, as always, the contingent America will send to the 1984 Olympics is very strong. The following includes the diets of some of the stars of those teams and the thoughts of their coaches, plus a look at the menu of the dining room of the Olympic Training Center in Colorado Springs. But first, some gastronomic words from the number one swimming hero of our last Summer Olympics.

If one were to conjure up a picture of "the ideal American athlete," chances are he would be **John Naber.** Six and a half feet tall (an even two meters), the twenty-four-year-old champion swimmer won four gold and one silver medal at Montreal in the 1976 Olympic Games. Chosen winner of the 1977 James E. Sullivan Award as the nation's Amateur Athlete of the Year, he also won twenty-five Amateur Athletic Union titles and claimed a record of ten National Collegiate Athletic Association individual titles during his four years as an All-American at the University of Southern California. Naber's world records for the one hundred and two hundred meter backstroke were so exceptional that they stood up years longer than usual in the arena of competitive swimming. As persuasive out of the pool as well as in, Naber is articulate not only about all sports but on many other topics—including food.

"I love to eat," Naber says. And when he's home in California, he likes to cook too. He hasn't had much of a chance lately though, because he has been on the road almost continually as an NBC swimming commentator and as an official spokesperson for the makers of Minute Maid products, urging support for the 1984 U.S. Olympic Team.

How did he stay in shape, and how does he continue to now that he is no longer swimming competitively? "I have no secrets, except that I love to eat all kinds of fresh vegetables and fruits and I drink tons of fruit juices." High protein diet? High carbohydrate? "Neither," says Naber. "Eat lots of everything, have a balanced diet and you'll do best."

Among his favorites are roast beef and spinach salad, pork chops and lasagna. For a quick energy boost, before or after working out in the pool, he recommends either a candy bar or orange juice, plain or mixed with other juices, such as his own creation, the Pasadena Flame, a blend of orange juice with apricot or papaya juice.

As he is a Californian, it's no surprise that Naber dotes on salads. A favorite meal is his own version of a chef's salad. He calls it a "super salad" and it includes anywhere from a dozen to twenty ingredients, depending on what's in the refrigerator. "Start with spinach, which has many valuable nutrients," he advises. "Then add as many kinds of lettuce as you can find— romaine, Boston, butter (anything but iceberg). To that, throw in sliced chicken, cubed cold roast beef, julienned strips of ham, shredded cold cuts, crumbled cooked bacon—just about any leftover meats or whatever you have on hand. Now it's time for a garden's bounty of vegetables—zucchini, carrots, mushrooms, blanched broccoli, cauliflower, green beans, new potatoes, cherry tomatoes and/or sprouts—all in bite-sized pieces." Naber likes fruit in his salad, too, usually chopped apples and oranges. For added nutrition, he tosses in sesame seeds and sometimes peanuts.

His favorite ranch-style dressing can be whipped up in a few minutes. It's a blend of buttermilk, mayonnaise, orange juice, heavy cream, and just a dash or two of red-hot pepper sauce. Naber's special salad secret: Top it off with crushed wheat thins instead of croutons. "They don't get soggy, no matter how much dressing you use."

When he's not traveling, Naber likes to get together with friends at his Pasadena apartment and concoct hot-weather drinks. "I do a variation on the old ice cream party. Depending on what's in season, I cut up bowls of fresh fruit—cantaloupes, strawberries, bananas, honeydew or crenshaw, bring out cracked ice, Minute Maid juices, and sparkling water, and everybody whirls a favorite combination. I call my specialty a Colorado Springs Cooler."

Here are some of Naber's most cherished recipes, starting with a breakfast potion suitably liquid for anyone whether or not they spend a good part of their day in water:

### LAST LAP ENERGY DRINK

Ingredients:
1 cup chilled orange juice from concentrate
2 tbsps. honey
2 tbsps. peanut butter
½ large, ripe banana

In blender container, combine all ingredients. Blend until smooth. Garnish with chopped peanuts, if desired.
Makes one serving (about ¾ cup)

## PASADENA FLAME

Ingredients:
1 cup orange juice
1 cup apricot or papaya juice
½ tsp. almond extract

Place ingredients in blender and mix on highest speed for ten seconds. Add ice cubes (two) and mix on medium speed for ten more seconds. Two Servings.

## RANCHO CALIFORNIA DRESSING

Ingredients:
1¼ cup orange juice
1 cup corn oil or other
   low cholesterol salad oil
1½ tsps. salt
1 clove garlic finely chopped
½ tsp. paprika
⅛ tsp. white pepper
1 tsp. chopped onion
1 tsp. celery seeds
1 tbsp. honey

Place all ingredients in a sealed jar and shake thirty times. Serve over salad. Makes two cups.

## JOHN'S BUTTERMILK-ORANGE SALAD DRESSING

Ingredients:
¼ cup frozen orange juice concentrate,
   thawed
¼ tsp. hot pepper sauce
Grated rind of one orange
¼ cup buttermilk
¼ cup mayonnaise
½ pint whipping cream,
   whipped

Combine first five ingredients and mix well. Fold this mixture into whipped cream. Makes about two and a half cups.

## OLYMPIC BOOSTER

Ingredients:
½ cup orange juice
2 tbsps. honey
1 tsp. wheat germ
2 ice cubes

Place all ingredients in blender and mix on high speed for ten seconds. When mixing a large batch, serve over cracked ice and float orange slices. Serves one.

## ORANGE GLAZED HAM KABOBS

Ingredients:
2 lbs. smoked ham, trimmed and cut into one inch cubes
2 large navel oranges, cut into wedges and each wedge halved
1 6-oz. can of frozen orange juice concentrate, undiluted
⅓ cup firmly packed brown sugar
Grated rind of a small lemon
¼ tsp. ground cloves

Spear ham cubes and half orange wedges on heatproof skewers. Combine remaining ingredients in small bowl and stir until well blended. Brush glaze over kabobs. Broil for five minutes. Brush with glaze again. Broil for one more minute. Turn and repeat for other side. If any glaze remains, heat and spoon over kabobs thinning glaze if necessary with water to a sauce consistency. Serves six to eight.

## COLORADO SPRINGS COOLER

Ingredients:
1 6-oz. can of frozen lemonade concentrate
6 strawberries
¼ medium cantaloupe

Place lemonade concentrate and two cans of water in blender. Mix on medium speed until well blended. Add fruit and blend for ten seconds at high speed. Serve over ice. Serves four.

The big U.S. hope in woman's swimming is the University of Florida's **Tracy Caulkins**. A young phenom who has matured into a full-fledged star, Caulkins has held more national titles (forty-seven) than any other swimmer in U.S. history. Winner of the Sullivan Award in 1978 at the tender age of fifteen, she was the youngest person ever to be so honored. Exceptionally versatile in a sport of specialists, Caulkins has held as many as fourteen world records in short and middle distance events in the free-style, breaststroke, backstroke, and, obviously, the individual medley. Going into the 1983–84 season, Caulkins had already broken American records an astounding fifty-nine times on her way to being a winner of the Broderick Cup as the top female college athlete in America.

A determined swimmer, Caulkins is equally positive about her diet: "The best advice is to try to eat balanced meals; this includes foods from the four food categories. I include whole grains like breads and cereals and stay away from junk food completely. My breakfast will be eggs, toast, and fruit—I love apples and oranges and bananas. I alternate this with cold cereal. Lunch is generally light, salads and sandwiches."

Dinner is Caulkin's heavy meal and it is very often red meat. "I find that meat gives me a great deal of energy and with this I will eat a lot of vegetables. And even though I like desserts, especially ice cream, I try to stay away from them as much as possible." The exception to this regime is the night before a meet. Then she will have spaghetti "for extra energy." The next day's preswim meal is not heavy. "Light, easily digestible foods such as French toast or eggs are important."

**Mary T. Meagher** is a world record holder in both the one hundred and two hundred meter butterfly. Another young superstar, according to **Bill Peak,** her coach at one of this country's premier AAU swimming clubs, the Lakeside Seahawks of Louisville, Kentucky, Meagher began to have a little trouble with her weight when she started college. The cure? "A high carbohydrate, low-fat diet got her to one thirty-six from one forty-six, at the same time allowing her to eat what she is comfortable with. The important thing is to stay away from junk food and for swimmers this is difficult. When the meet is over at ten o'clock at night that's the only thing to eat."

To avoid running short of fuel and getting the munchies when there isn't anything nutritious available, Coach Peak recommends using the powder diets such as the Cambridge program as a supplement to, not instead of, eating regular meals. "Swimmers cannot afford to be low on energy. They also can't afford to be heavy, although some feel that it is the higher degree of body fat that keeps women more buoyant, therefore on an equal par with men." The following is a diet that Meagher follows for a few days when she wants to get her weight down:

*Mary T. Meagher's Quick Weight-Loss Diet*

Breakfast is a cereal such as corn flakes with lots of bran and a piece of whole grain toast, alternating with poached eggs on toast. All meals are supplemented with a banana, an apple, an orange, or a grapefruit.

Lunch is a peanut butter ("be sure to get the natural kind, without hydrogenated oil") or an egg salad or a tuna fish sandwich on whole wheat bread. A good high-protein substitute is soup made from either pinto or navy beans.

Dinner combines low-fat protein chicken or fish (red meat on occasion) with any green vegetable—good ones are string beans, peas, and spinach—along with a baked potato ("the only time potatoes become fattening is when you add butter or sour cream; otherwise they are an ideal food"). Dessert is always fruit.

Richard Quick, head coach of the University of Texas Women's Swimming Team, is also the personal coach of **Ambrose "Rowdy" Gaines IV** (nicknamed after the Clint Eastwood character in the old TV western series *Rawhide*), whom he first met while he was the head coach of the Auburn University Men's Swimming Team. As a the holder of the world's record in the one hundred-meter freestyle, Gaines earned the title of world's fastest human (waterborne division). Coach Quick believes that many athletes overlook nutrition as an important part of performance. "There are some overwhelming misconceptions among young athletes," he says. "Too much red meat and too many dairy products are not good. Athletes should also replace ordinary white bread and packaged cereals with the more nutritious whole grain types and should eat more complex carbohydrates."

Gaines follows his diet advice as well as his swimming tips: "When I wake up at five for a six o'clock practice, I'll just have a piece of fruit and maybe some yogurt. After the workout I'll have a real breakfast. I'm what they call a pancakeaholic, I love them with pure maple syrup. I alternate these with French toast or waffles, and some days I'll have a bowl of hot oatmeal with brown sugar, bacon, and a few glasses of fruit juice, grape or orange. I drink nothing whatsoever with caffeine in it. I might also add a half a grapefruit or a half a cantaloupe."

Lunch is generally a light meal; just a sandwich or a bowl of spaghetti. He then swims from three to five. Dinner is the largest meal of the day. "I'm like my favorite baseball player, Wade Boggs of the Boston Red Sox [who won the Major League's batting title in 1983 by a wide margin], I can eat chicken seven nights a week. I bake it or broil it or fry it; cooked any way, it's wonderful." With this he'll have a good salad plus vegetables, broccoli or string beans, along with spaghetti or potatoes, and lots of fruit for dessert (peaches, plums, oranges, or grapefruit —he is, after all, from Florida). "I generally eat a good mix of protein and carbohydrates but two days before every meet, I stop eating all red meat and just have lighter foods like fish or chicken and load up on spaghetti, lasagna, and fruit. I find this works best for me."

While Gaines has been able to exchange white bread for whole wheat, he cannot manage to give up Double Stuffed Oreos. If you swim ten miles a day, some things you can get away with.

**Steve Lundquist** of Southern Methodist University, a holder of the one hundred yard breaststroke world record plus his share of the NCAA two hundred and four hundred yard medley relay records, was voted the U.S. Male Swimmer of the Year in

196

1982. Lundquist's stroke may differ from Gaines's, but his diet is very much the same.

For his preswim meal, Lundquist generally has pancakes, eggs, and peach halves. His coach at SMU, **George McMillan**, recommends anything you can digest quickly, such as spaghetti and lasagna, but especially pancakes and scrambled eggs. "Stay away from the fried foods," he suggests, "scrambled and soft boiled are the best. Peach halves go well with eggs and pancakes. You should eat about four hours before a swim. In this way, the blood needed to digest the meal will have already done its thing, will be ready to oxygenate the muscles. The food will also now be in the bloodstream."

One of Naber's teammates at the 1976 Olympic Games in Montreal, **Wendy Boglioli**, helped the American four by one hundred-meter freestyle relay team set a world record and capture the gold medal. She also earned a bronze medal by setting an American record in the one hundred meter butterfly. Outside the pool, Boglioli has donated her time to a number of organizations. She is currently a member of the Athletes' Advisory Council to the U.S. Olympic Committee, an adviser to the Women's Sports Foundation, and a member of the New Jersey Governor's Council on Physical Fitness. She also does volunteer work for the N.J. Special Olympics program.

What's more, Boglioli is a full-time homemaker, mother, and author-to-be. In her spare time, she is writing her autobiography.

During one of the infrequent breaks in her hectic schedule, Boglioli outlined her diet, which is basically a mixture of simple and complex carbohydrates built around many small meals and snacks rather than the usual three squares. Her snacks were often snack bars or candy for quick energy; while this may seem unorthodox, it is interesting that in recent studies done on how quickly different foods are converted into blood sugar, Mars bars ranked better (i.e., slower) than honey, carrots, bread, and corn flakes.

**Don Gambril** has been selected as the top American men's swimming coach by both the U.S. Olympic Committee and his peers, being the President of the American Swimming Coaches Association. Besides coaching Harvard's *Crimson,* and for more than ten years, Alabama's *Crimson Tide,* one additional other thing makes Coach Gambril see red—poor dietary habits. Coach Gambril has a special reason why he believes in a nutritious diet. He recently, at quite a young age, underwent cardiovascular bypass surgery and strongly believes that it is never too early (or too late) to get on a good program.

"Athletes and everyone else would benefit from two simple rules: Eat less red meat and lean towards raw fruits, vegetables, and whole grains. The traditional American breakfast of eggs, bacon, and fried foods should be replaced by whole grain cereals, fruits, and skim milk. Bananas are good as they are high in potassium, as are citrus fruits, and raisins which provide energy (and iron as well). Stay away from all processed sugars, including the sugar coated cold cereals. The best kinds are Shredded Wheat or plain oatmeal without sugar or salt. Be careful of some packaged cereals; they contain as much salt as you would find in a bag of potato chips."

Coach Gambril recommends taking a good multiple and a B complex vitamin and a mineral tablet at breakfast, two hundred to four hundred units of vitamin E, and a thousand milligrams of vitamin C taken daily spread over two or three doses (this is especially necessary if you are under stress).

"Snack all you want, but do it on the right foods; a piece of fruit or some raw vegetables. Peaches, apples, and bananas are good snacks and nutritious food. Lunch can be tuna packed in water. Meat once a day in the form of chicken or fish (I believe it is better to have this protein for lunch because after dinner you are less active) along with vegetables and fruit, and if necessary a slice of whole grain bread. Beware of red meat. Even lean, it contains about nineteen percent fat. Fat has about nine calories per gram. And something as innocent as a quarter pounder is total fat content. In fact, the average person should not have more than fifteen to twenty percent fat in their diets. Excellent vegetables are broccoli, cabbage, and cauliflower, all high in vitamin C (hold the cheese sauce, however).

"Dinner would be chicken breasts or baked or grilled fish

(if not had at lunchtime) with a baked potato and vegetables such as cabbage or squash. Add a large salad using a dressing made with a corn oil and seasoned with garlic powder. You may have something such as chili, but make it with turkey instead of red meat. A good snack throughout the day is a small serving of Grape Nuts. This is a chewy cereal that is filling and satisfying."

In addition to his sample menu, Coach Gambril has the following tips:

• Use little salt, no processed sugars, little fat, little cholesterol (interestingly enough, even shrimp are high in cholesterol).
• A wonderful way to cook food is in a crock pot where it cooks in its own natural juices. A great crock-pot dinner consists of navy beans, turnips, potatoes, celery, carrots, onion, celery leaves, garlic powder, pepper, nonfat chicken bouillon, over brown rice.
• If you're hungry during the afternoon, try a fruit shake. Put four or five strawberries into a blender, add a banana, skim milk, three or four ice cubes, and blend.
• Try substituting raisins in things in place of sugar, in oatmeal for example.
• Look for fat content on the labels—it should be only about 1 percent.
• Spaghetti (without meat sauce) and waffles (without butter or margarine) are good carbohydrate pregame meals. If buying frozen waffles, however, look for the ones without additives made from whole wheat flour and nonfat buttermilk.
• Use egg whites instead of egg yolks in most dishes (even an omelette can be whipped up with two egg whites and one yolk).
• In extended competitions you should eat something in between that is a good source of energy, raisins for example.
• Eat more whole grains, raw fruits, and vegetables, and drink more fruit juices (orange juice usually contains too much acid). Always buy juices with no sugar added.
• The last point to remember is that most active swimmers need four thousand to five thousand calories daily.

The U.S. training center for all the 1984 Olympics is in Colorado Springs in Colorado. At the training center the athletes spend a considerable amount of time educating themselves about diet and finding out what works best for them.

**Dr. Casey Clarke,** director of sports medicine for the Olympic Training Center, says: "Nutrition is important; it should be taken seriously, including the appreciation for the balance of nutrients and sufficient calories. Nutrition does not make the athlete. However, the athlete can support the training it takes to become a great athlete better if he is well fed."

In fact, says **Dr. Peter van Handle,** head of the sports Physiology Department there, "most of the questions asked by the young athletes at the center are concerned with nutrition—what is the proper vitamin dosage, how to replace the fluids lost in competition, the need for protein, and the benefits of vegetarianism."

At the center, meals are conceived by **Francis Veuthy,** director of the dining halls. Here is a sampling of some of the choices on the menu. First, the salad bar.

*The Olympic Training Center Salad Bar*

mixed tossed salad
blue cheese dressing
low calorie French dressing
French dressing
Italian dressing
Thousand island dressing
vinegar & oil dressing
croutons
leaf spinach
alfalfa sprouts
bean sprouts
egg noodles
bacon pieces
garbanzo beans
salami
bologna

macaroni salad
cole slaw
pickle spears
mayonnaise
ketchup
mustard
Gulden's mustard
fruit yogurt
plain yogurt
cottage cheese
kidney beans
raw fresh broccoli
raw fresh cauliflower
fresh mushrooms
pickled beets
peanut butter

| | |
|---|---|
| boiled eggs | jelly |
| American cheese | horseradish |
| Swiss cheese | relish tray |
| lemon wedges | fruits |
| potato salad | dessert |
| Perrier water | |

*Two Weeks at the Olympic Training Center*

## First Week

### Sunday

*Breakfast*  fruit juices
scrambled eggs
hash-brown potatoes
choice of dry cereals
stewed prunes
toast and jelly

*Lunch*  assorted cold meat platter with potato salad
rice pilaf
buttered peas

*Dinner*  roast round of beef, au jus
baked potato
buttered cauliflower

### Monday

*Breakfast*  fruit juices
French-dip waffles, syrup
bacon
choice of dry cereals
oranges, apples, bananas
muffins

*Lunch*  hamburger
Italian-style zucchini

*Dinner*          carrots Vichy
                  ice cream

## Tuesday

*Breakfast*       fruit juices
                  scrambled eggs
                  choice of dry cereals
                  oranges, apples, bananas
                  banana bread

*Lunch*           baked meat loaf-Creole sauce
                  whipped potatoes
                  mixed vegetables

*Dinner*          bar-b-qued chicken
                  potato triangles
                  buttered Brussels sprouts

## Wednesday

*Breakfast*       fruit juices
                  French toast, syrup
                  choice of dry cereals
                  oranges, apples, bananas

*Lunch*           teriyaki steak
                  buttered sliced carrots
                  ice cream

*Dinner*          roast pork
                  whipped potatoes
                  corn on the cob
                  fruit

## Thursday

*Breakfast*       fruit juices
                  scrambled eggs

hash-brown potatoes
choice of dry cereals
oranges, apples, bananas
toast and jelly

*Lunch*   boiled brisket of corned beef and
cabbage
potatoes
buttered cut green beans
pie

*Dinner*   Swiss steak
cut wax beans
oven-browned potatoes
ice cream

## Friday

*Breakfast*   fruit juices
buttermilk pancakes, syrup
choice of dry cereals
oranges, apples, bananas
muffins

*Lunch*   baked codfish Mornay
Italian spaghetti with meat sauce
garlic bread
buttered succotash

*Dinner*   grilled round steak
buttered cauliflower
rice and raisin pudding

## Saturday

*Breakfast*   fruit juices
scrambled eggs
choice of dry cereals
oranges, apples, bananas
toast and jelly

| | |
|---|---|
| *Lunch* | beef enchiladas<br>Spanish rice<br>sour cabbage<br>corn O'Brien<br>ice cream |
| *Dinner* | veal cutlet Parmesan<br>buttered egg noodles<br>buttered green peas |

## Second Week

### Sunday

| | |
|---|---|
| *Breakfast* | fruit juices<br>French toast, syrup<br>choice of dry cereals<br>oranges, apples, bananas<br>blueberry muffins |
| *Lunch* | baked chicken<br>whipped potatoes<br>corn niblets<br>tropical fruit |
| *Dinner* | assorted cold meat<br>potato salad<br>mashed potatoes<br>baby lima beans |

### Monday

| | |
|---|---|
| *Breakfast* | fruit juices<br>scrambled eggs<br>choice of dry cereals<br>oranges, apples, bananas<br>toast and jelly |
| *Lunch* | beef stew with garden vegetables<br>cold turkey sandwich |

scalloped potatoes
Brussels sprouts
ice cream

*Dinner*      hamburger on a bun
green peas
pie

## Tuesday

*Breakfast*      fruit juices
French-dip waffles
choice of dry cereals
oranges, apples, bananas
banana bread

*Lunch*      ravioli with meat sauce
garlic bread
hash-brown potatoes
cut green beans
brownies

*Dinner*      grilled pork chops
apple sauce
au gratin potatoes
corn on the cob
ice cream

## Wednesday

*Breakfast*      fruit juices
scrambled eggs
choice of dry cereals
oranges, apples, bananas
toast and jelly

*Lunch*      oven-browned potatoes
green peas

*Dinner*　　　　brisket of corned beef and cabbage
　　　　　　　boiled potatoes
　　　　　　　sliced carrots
　　　　　　　cake

## Thursday

*Breakfast*　　　fruit juices
　　　　　　　buttermilk pancakes, syrup
　　　　　　　choice of dry cereals
　　　　　　　oranges, apples, bananas
　　　　　　　bran muffins

*Lunch*　　　　Italian spaghetti with meat sauce
　　　　　　　garlic bread
　　　　　　　baked codfish Mornay
　　　　　　　cut wax beans

*Dinner*　　　　steak teriyaki
　　　　　　　baked potatoes
　　　　　　　buttered cauliflower
　　　　　　　rice and raisin pudding

## Friday

*Breakfast*　　　fruit juices
　　　　　　　scrambled eggs
　　　　　　　hash-brown potatoes
　　　　　　　choice of dry cereals
　　　　　　　oranges, apples, bananas
　　　　　　　toast and jelly

*Lunch*　　　　assorted cold meat plate with potato salad
　　　　　　　cut green beans
　　　　　　　apple pie

*Dinner*　　　　fish
　　　　　　　green peas

## Saturday

*Breakfast*       fruit juices
French toast
hash-brown potatoes
choice of dry cereals
oranges, apples, bananas

*Lunch*       Swiss steak
mashed potatoes
mixed vegetables
ice cream

*Dinner*       chicken chop suey with Chinese egg noodles
brown rice
Brussels sprouts
brownies

# CHAPTER TEN

# Skiing

Both downhill and cross-country skiing are comparatively young competitive sports. In fact, the very first downhill, or Alpine, races date only to 1911 (in Switzerland, of course). And cross-country, or Nordic, skiing has fostered a following outside its traditional Scandinavian homeland only in the last decade. But skiing of one sort or another is considerably older than even the original Olympics. Archeological finds in several countries date skiing hunters and warriors back forty-five hundred years, with suggestions of much earlier antecedents. Its role in Norwegian and Swedish history is commemorated by two marathon races of historic proportions. The Birkebeiner (which now has an American namesake in the northwest corner of Wisconsin) covers the thirty-five kilometer route taken in 1206 by the saviors of Norway's infant King Haakon Haakonsson; while the granddaddy of cross-country marathons, the Vasaloppet, retraces the whopping eighty-five and a half kilometers (versus Pheidippides's modest forty-two kilometers on foot) taken by Gustav Vasa and his men in 1522 to overcome Danish forces in Sweden.

The history of skiing in this country is generally associated with Jon Torsteinson Rue, better known as Snowshoe Thompson. The Thompson is from his stepfather, but the Snowshoe can only be because they didn't have a better name for skis back in the 1860's, 1870's, and 1880's when he was the mailman in the

High Sierras. It was around this time that modern skis were being developed in the Telemark region of Norway (whence Snowshoe Thompson emigrated when he was a precocious two-year-old). They revolutionized the sport and were the springboard to the maneuverability that created Alpine skiing shortly thereafter, with the downhill disciplines reaching their first zenith in the 1920's and 1930's following such developments as the Jungfrau Railway and the introduction of ski tows and lifts.

The dash and danger of Alpine skiing soon eclipsed its Nordic progenitor in popularity. The Olympics and World Cup races and personalities—not to mention the legendary bronzed ski instructors and bunnies—captured the public's imagination here and abroad as modern technology permitted easier and more comfortable access to the high slopes. But just as the marathon has caught up with the hundred yard dash in track, cross-country skiing has made a strong comeback in the age of fitness and cardiovascular conditioning.

Here are some of the thoughts and diets of champions of both sports as well as from their coaches and trainers, plus a special section prepared by The Shaklee Corporation, the giant food-supplement company that has been the official nutrition consultants to the U.S. Ski Team since 1981.

# Alpine

**Jean-Claude Killy** is still probably the best-known name in skiing. His Olympic Grand Slam in 1968 is every Alpine skier's dream. Being able to dominate in all three events, the Downhill, Slalom, and Grand Slalom, requires an extraordinary combination of strength, in both the legs and upper body, agility, and flexibility. Some of the greatest Alpine skiers, Sweden's slalom king Ingemar Stenmark, for example, won't even compete in all three events.

Killy based his skiing diet on protein, which he felt helped to fight the cold, but without too much red meat. "During the winter my heavy meal is fresh vegetable soup, followed by brown rice or spaghetti and a local unpasteurized cheese. I drink about half a gallon of mineral water a day, and eat only whole-grain bread with a delicious specialty of my native French Alps —honey drawn from select combs without boiling. When I come back from a trip after having overindulged, I go on this diet for a few days: Breakfast is walnuts and almonds plus some dried fruit (apricots, raisins, figs, and dried bananas) and lunch and dinner are raw carrots with fresh olive oil and brown rice with soy sauce."

Since retiring from ski racing, Killy has taken up France's national sport—*cyclisme*—bicycle racing. "As in skiing, protein foods like chicken and fish are important. I also carry a high energy drink with me that consists of protein powder, a pint of raw milk, two egg yolks, and a banana."

The most familiar name in women's skiing in America over the last several years is **Cindy Nelson.** Cindy, at twenty-eight, is the senior member of the U.S. Women's Ski Team and has been a force to contend with in World Cup skiing since her teens. At five feet, six inches, she weighs between 135 and 140 pounds in order to maintain her power. Breakfast for Nelson is light toast or cereal with one cup of coffee with milk. Lunch is generally a protein, such as chicken or fish, with lots of fresh vegetables. After a day on the slopes, dinner is generally large and balanced, with some protein, vegetables, salad, and dessert. She drinks orange juice from time to time but finds that the drink that she does best on is beer. "Beer is full of minerals and I will have a couple of them a day with meals.

"In the summer I have to watch my weight, as I have a tendency to bulk up. In the winter, however, it is difficult for me to keep weight on, as you burn up a lot more calories staying warm. In addition, on tour in Europe we often have trouble getting fresh food. You really begin to miss fresh vegetables and green salads. I just watch what I eat and try to eat balanced meals. In Italy at least there is generally fresh pasta. I think in part because of the lack of fresh food, I used to have a problem with colds, but now that I get more sleep and take vitamin C supplements regularly I find that they are not so common anymore."

Nelson was interviewed while at a training camp in one of America's great skiing centers, Hawaii. After rising at six in the morning and starting with running distances and sprints, swimming, weight lifting, and paddling outrigger canoes, she finally stopped at four for a lunch break. And what was it? Just half an omelette!

Training Nelson along with the rest of the Women's Team is **John Atkins.** "We are on the road nine months a year. To give the women stability I try to emphasize a well-balanced diet. Vegetarianism just doesn't work out. I think breakfast should be substantial: fresh fruit, such as a half grapefruit, cereal, preferably something on the order of granola, plus whole grain bread. It also very important to stay hydrated with orange or grapefruit juice, and the women like to have a cup of yogurt for breakfast as well.

"Lunch in Europe is a salad along with carbohydrates, potatoes, or pasta. Be sure to have things baked as opposed to fried, and try to get lean cuts of meat or fish. If you have chicken, take the skin off as you really don't need that fat. There is no dessert for lunch. Dinner is similar to lunch in the U.S. It includes whole grains, vegetables, and fresh fruits.

"Stateside at our training table we like to offer two or three varieties of things. Breakfast can be dry cereals, eggs, and a starch, like pancakes. Lunch is sandwiches and soup, while dinner is meat, potatoes, salads, and vegetables. It is important during summer training to drink at least six glasses of fluids daily.

"During winter it's a bit different. You should have smaller breakfasts and not eat a large meal within two hours of a competition (two hours instead of the usual four—in the cold weather you burn up calories more quickly). High-energy bars make a good midday snack. If you are tired, increase your liquids and take more carbohydrates for the next day."

Atkins also has advice for the rest of us: "There are a couple of things that weekend skiers should take note of. You do not need a whole lot of food. You can stay warm by drinking liquids and having high-energy snacks. You might simply want to eat another slice of toast for breakfast, for example, if you want to increase your carbohydrates. Take a good multi-vitamin supplement and stay away from junk food, which can take away more than it gives. It is also a good idea to take a time-release vitamin C which we have found helps avoid colds. About five hundred milligrams in the morning seems to work the best."

**Toper Haggerman,** the coach of the U.S. Men's Ski Team, including of course their superstar Phil Mahre, is in general agreement with his colleagues. "Basically I recommend a sound and balanced diet for my athletes, but the great amount of traveling that we do puts a tremendous burden on them. It is most difficult in Europe when we are almost constantly going from one World Cup match to another. When we are abroad this is a sampling of the kinds of foods that are offered. After rising about six-thirty for early stretching exercises, breakfast is good sized, with cheese and breads, fruit, fruit juice, and dry cereal with milk. Yogurt is also good for breakfast. We often do not have eggs and everything is generally on the cold side. During the day dehydration is probably the most common thing that sneaks up on athletes, so I recommend that all my men carry a thermos with herb teas and juices, plus fruit bars for quick energy. Lunches in Europe are rather large and tend to include salad, soup, potatoes, and vegetables (peas, corn, carrots, and green beans) in addition to some meats; pork, beef, and veal, which is very popular in Alpine countries, are the usual main courses. Snacks are yogurt and cookies. The point is that I don't want my athletes to lose weight. We take a scale with us— always. Dinner is similar to lunch, though in Europe lunches are generally larger.

"Basically, my advice for skiers is that there is nothing magical about diets. A good diet for skiers should consist of fifty-five percent carbohydrates, thirty-five percent fat and the rest proteins. A general rule of thumb is that the body uses carbohydrates and fat for energy, but proteins for muscle tissue and growth. Skiers actually train harder in summer, so they need more carbohydrates. As calorie usage increases, so should the caloric intake. But if you're gaining weight, you're probably taking in too many. Don't be a glutton!

"On the other hand, a lot of people get carried away with

carbohydrate loading. In our sport, I recommend that they be increased prior to events but without depleting before. That just throws the system off. Start four to six days before a competition to increase the carbohydrates. The best ones are starches—breads, pancakes, pastas, and cereals, not the simple sugars. Also remember what doesn't settle and keep track of those foods to be avoided.

"Our men are very conscious of good nutrition. They generally find that dinner the night before is the most important meal. In the evening, I recommend a special fruit whip to give them more energy for the next day: Put some fresh orange juice into a blender, add fresh strawberries and vanilla ice cream for a delicious drink." Finally, Haggerman's advice for those who have a long trip to the slopes: "If you're tired from travel, fill up with liquids, water or orange juice. Do not drink alcohol (beer is okay) and take vitamin C and B complex."

## Nordic

The king of cross-country is clearly **Bill Koch.** It all started when, as a relative youngster of twenty (by Nordic standards), Bill won the Silver Medal in the thirty kilometer race at the 1976 Olympics in Austria. It was in 1980, though, that he reached the heights, winning four international races, and becoming the first American ever to win cross-country's World Cup.

For Koch, diet is important, and he tries to eat well-balanced meals. On the other hand, he is not terribly strict about his diet. The only basic rules that he follows are no junk food and plenty of sleep.

Breakfast is pancakes or eggs or a hot cereal, such as oatmeal, and orange juice. He drinks skim milk but no coffee or tea. He uses common sense in everything and though he feels that if you are eating properly, vitamins are not really necessary, he takes a multiple vitamin supplement every day on the theory that they "can't hurt." Lunch is something light, like a sandwich and a salad. Dinner is the heavier meal and it will be high in carbohydrates, with vegetables and a small portion of meat. "I will never eat a large steak, for example. Casseroles are a good meal, with beans and other vegetables plus a little chicken. I'll always have a salad as well." Dessert is generally fruit, his favorite being bananas, apples, and pears. Ice cream is Koch's weak spot, but to get around that he bought an ice-cream maker so he at least knows exactly what ingredients are going into it. Koch's diet stays with him all through his travels. "I always stay away from junk. In fact, in the Communist countries where there is not a whole lot of choice, I bring food like dried fruit to keep me going."

If he is racing fifty kilometers, Koch will eat more potatoes the night before, and perhaps eat more carbohydrates starting a few days prior to the race. If it is a long race, sometimes he will "feed" along the way. He drinks, mostly water, at intervals, and at times will have something like a banana. The important thing is to be prepared so that the main event is within one's capabilities, or as Koch puts it, "Racing should be nothing to get upset about." And from someone who has raced cross-country in deep snow for eighty-nine kilometers (equivalent to fifty-five miles) in about four hours, he shouldn't get upset about anything.

**Mike Gallagher** is the coach of the U.S. Men's Cross-Country Ski Team, and he has come to several conclusions about diet in relation to his cross-country skiers. "In the first place, in a cold environment you burn more calories than you would in a warm one. However, most diets are too high in fat, especially from animal protein sources like red meat, whole milk, butter, and cheese.

"One of the first things that I impress on my athletes is that they should drink plenty of liquids. A trademark, in fact, of my men is that they never travel anywhere without water. My maxim is that it's even more important than their ski boots. Europeans drink more water in general, and now Americans are catching up.

"We travel just as much as the Alpine skiers, and are similarly at the mercy of what is available in hotels. We simply look at the menu like everyone else. The only special requests that we make of men in fifty kilometer races are that two days before the competition they go high on carbohydrates, rice and potatoes, and cut down on meat. Another problem is that we do not find the "Continental breakfast" adequate for our athletes. Ideally, a diet for cross-country skiing should be a choice of cereals, both hot and cold, and soft boiled eggs. No bacon or sausage, however. Milk or water, tea, or coffee. Some of the athletes find that they take coffee as a "feed" during the race. They are normally light coffee drinkers, and when competing, after about twenty or forty kilometers, they take six to eight ounces of coffee with a little sugar.

"When eating bread, we always ask for the whole grain types. This is where Europe is superior. Many of the hotels we regularly stay at have fresh homemade breads. The women usually have two slices with breakfast and the men three or four with butter.

"Lunch should be something simple, such as a sandwich and soup or a salad. The sandwich should consist of cheese or turkey, staying away from the greasy meats. There should always be a green salad with oil and vinegar dressing. Dinner should be the heavy meal with meat or fish (most of the athletes prefer meat) along with rice, noodles, or vegetables. In Scandinavia, Austria, Switzerland, and Germany there are usually no vegetables served, simply meat and potatoes, and in the Eastern bloc countries we have gone so far as to bring our own food. The best part of the meals there is the breads, but the food is greasy in general. We bring in Shaklee supplements along with their protein drinks. For dessert, we almost always try to have fresh fruit if it's available. The best is oranges (for vitamin C and fluids) and with apples (for roughage) and bananas (potassium) as close seconds.

"The weekend cross-country skier, however, will not burn up the three thousand to five thousand calories a day that our athletes do. Here are some recommendations for everyone who is interested in the sport: Eat conservatively. We don't need as much food as you think. Show the same amount of discipline in eating as you do in training. Try to eat balanced meals, staying away from fat but including a modest amount of meat. Athletes sometimes have the same problem that others have, they eat too much. This causes them to lose sleep and gives them trouble with digestion. Even one full spoon of honey in a cup of tea is too much. Since water is so important for our athletes, we tell them that too much sugar in the stomach will slow down their ability to absorb liquids. If we eat anything sweet, we should therefore consume a lot of water to offset the sugar imbalance. Stick with the liquids that are low in sugar, those are the ones that are most easily assimilated."

### The Shaklee Dietary Program for the U.S. Ski Team

The following is a report prepared especially for this book by Shaklee.

For the U.S. Ski Team, usually pressed for time and funds, nutrition used to take last place. While traveling to ski events in foreign countries, athletes ate whatever was available. In one European hotel, the coaches recall, there was nothing to be had in the morning except wine and bread—clearly not a breakfast for champions.

Four years ago, however, U.S. Ski Team physicians realized that their athletes needed a nutritional boost. Nutrition, the doctors thought, might help the skiers resist infection, heal wounds, and improve performance. They turned to The Shaklee Corporation for help. In 1981, the Ski Team's Sports Medicine Council named Shaklee as the "official nutrition consultant to the U.S. Ski Team."

Under the direction of Drs. James Scala and James Whittam, Shaklee's Health Sciences staff nutritionists and dietitians began investigating the special nutritional needs of these athletes. As a start, they spent over a year collecting data in conjunction with Stanford University's Heart Disease Prevention Program and Dr. William Haskell to determine the athlete's baseline levels of caloric expenditures and nutritional intakes. They had them keep complete three-day food diaries at four periods throughout the year: One at training camp, one at U.S. competition, one at European competition, and one when the skiers were at home.

The data collected reveals some astounding facts. First of all, these athletes, while training, consume almost twice the amount of calories per day as the average individual. For men this was about five thousand and for women approximately thirty-five hundred. The National Academy of Sciences Recommended Energy Intakes for men and women are approximately twenty-eight hundred and twenty-one hundred calories respectively. Secondly, like most American diets, theirs were extremely high in fat at the expense of carbohydrates. Carbohydrates have nutrients especially needed by athletes since they are a key fuel for aerobic capacity and are important in building glycogen stores for endurance. The difference between the ideal and actual proportions of nutrients is shown in the diagram. Nutritionists and specialists in this area would recommend a balance of nutrients of 15 percent protein, less than 30 percent fat, and not more than 55 percent carbohydrates.

In a second study conducted in conjunction with Dr. Emily Haynes at Florida State University, the iron stores of about twenty Nordic endurance women were checked over a twelve-month competition period. This data revealed that the iron stores of these athletes, who travel from location to location, fluctuated, especially as altitude changed. In addition, there was a statistically significant decrease in the iron stores of these women during the long competition period. Whether this was due to poor diet or to an exercise factor known as sports anemia is unclear. Nevertheless, it warrants an increase in iron-rich foods. The Haynes study also found that those skiers who were provided with a multi-vitamin/multi-mineral supplement containing eighteen milligrams of iron (100 percent USRDA) also fluctuated due to the altitude effect but maintained their iron stores at a higher level than the control group. This indicated that these athletes need an iron supplement when they compete and travel on a typical schedule that does not allow for well-planned meals.

As far as other nutritional supplements are concerned, a thorough review of the results of other studies and scientific writings resulted in the following findings (as set forth in greater detail in Dr. Scala's article in March 1981 in the *Journal of the United States Ski Coaches Association*):

1. Since endurance training burns up about twice the normal caloric usage, it is reasonable to expect that the need for all of the micronutrients is also at least doubled.
2. The body might excrete extra thiamin and ascorbic acid during training. Whether this is because the need is lower or because it is a necessary consequence of glycogen mobilization is unclear. But in any case, the thiamin should be replaced to maintain balance, since reduced thiamin can lead to early fatigue and lower endurance of the athletes within weeks, even though normally deficiencies only show after months.
3. In addition to the losses referred to above, some studies indicate

## CALORIE DISTRIBUTION OF SKIERS

### IDEAL

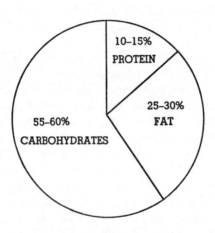

### ACTUAL

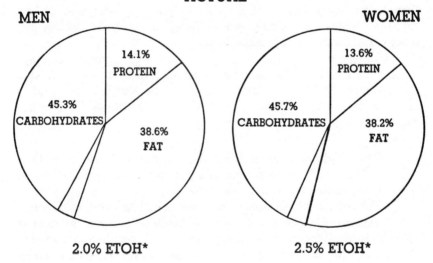

*Alcohol and related products

that vitamin C requirements are elevated by extreme athletic stress and higher body temperatures. These tend to go hand in hand anyway, since body temperature tends to increase under intense stress. At least one expert feels that hard training requires about five hundred milligrams daily, almost ten times the normal USRDA.

4. Even at only 15 percent of caloric intake, protein would be about 220 grams (one-half pound) daily. This large amount should be expected to increase calcium excretion in addition. More is lost through perspiration. Therefore, there is a good case for more than a doubling of the RDA for calcium. Similarly, the high levels of protein assimilation require extra riboflavin.

5. Vitamin E may be the most undervalued micronutrient for athletes. It is important for its anti-oxidant qualities. Studies of rigorous athletic performance suggest a need as high as twelve hundred IU per day—one hundred times the RDA.

6. The one contraindication comes from niacin. Nicotinic acid has been found to inhibit the mobilization of free fatty acids. This could impede optimum performance by forcing more rapid consumption of glycogen by the muscles.

As a result of this data, Shaklee nutritionists developed a series of educational lectures and literature on proper nutrition to help instill better eating habits in both the coaches and the athletes.

In preparation for the Winter Olympics, Dr. Whittam, at the request of James Page, director of the U.S. Nordic Team, visited Sarajevo at the World Cup games in February 1983, to personally evaluate the U.S. team's nutritional program. A diet survey was taken during the week of competition when the athletes were eating typical Yugoslavian food at a major hotel. This survey emphatically confirmed what the earlier studies had shown: the diets were as high as 45 to 47 percent fat, with 17 percent protein and the remainder in carbohydrates. Basic fruits and vegetables taken for granted in the U.S. were lacking. According to Mr. Page, this type of diet is quite typical when the team travels in Europe, especially in the Eastern bloc countries. This points to a real problem. Athletes, to compete successfully, need to anticipate different types of foods in various countries. Some athletes now carry an extra suitcase full of packaged products or fruits and vegetables to ensure that they fulfill their sensory requirements as well as their nutrutional needs.

At the Olympics, the situation was quite different. A full training table was available for the athletes. Dr. Whittam and Dr. Edward Hixson, the Nordic Ski Team physician, had met with the organizing committee of the Winter Games, Prim. Dr. Slobodan, sports medicine specialist/Chief of Medical Science, XIV Olympic Winter Games, Sarajevo '84, and Mr. Dreso, operations manager, United Agriculture Trade & Industry, Sarajevo, Yugoslavia, and were able to obtain a list of the foods that were to be available at the Olympic Village. Taking no chances in efforts to optimize the athlete's diet, they had Shaklee Health Sciences nutritionists and dietitians compile a series of guidelines for the coaches and athletes. These guidelines included varying calorie levels and carbohydrate levels. More usefully, these were further broken down among the foods that are available on a given day at the Olympic Village. An example of this is shown in the chart on pages 222–223.

Another concern of these athletes, especially those competing in endurance events such as the thirty kilometer and fifty kilometer cross-country events, is fluid replacement. Many have their own antidotal formulas and secrets. The American College of Sports Medicine, in its *Position Statement on Prevention of Heat Injuries During Distance Running*, recommends that fluids for water replacement should contain not more than 2.5 percent glucose, to give a little boost to blood sugar levels without overly slowing down the absorption of the water into the system—or even causing water to leave the muscles in order for the stomach to dilute the sugar from the drink. Similarly, they should have less than ten milliequivalents (mEq) (.025 percent) sodium (salt) and five mEq (.02 percent) potassium per liter. In most cases, this means careful mixing of the commercially available thirst-quenching drinks and, as a guideline, often diluting the formulation by half to achieve these desired levels.

According to Drs. Whittam and Scala, these efforts should optimize nutrition for these athletes to the point where it becomes a secondary concern. After all, their primary concern should be the race at hand. And for those not actually racing, here are Shakelee's tips for weekend skiers:

• Cross-country skiing is more demanding and involves a higher caloric output.
• The typical American diet is not optimal for weekend athletes because it's too high in fat. Forty-percent of our diet is fat and 43 percent is carbohydrate. Thirty percent fat and 50 percent carbohydrates would be a better balance for skiers.

• Carbohydrates should be the foods of the weekend skier's diet. Carbohydrates are stored in the muscles as glycogen. Glycogen is the primary source of muscle energy. Studies show that people who are injured on the slopes have low or depleted glycogen stores. Their muscles are weak and the result is injury.

• For better performance on the slopes, here are some guidelines for the weekend skier:

1. Dinner the night before should abound in complex carbohydrates; pasta, rice, potatoes, macaroni, and breads are ideal.
2. Breakfast should also contain plenty of complex carbohydrates. Choose pancakes and oatmeal instead of bacon and eggs.
3. Snacks on the slopes should not be simple sugary carbohydrates like candy bars. Muffins, crackers, popcorn, and crusty breads are better choices.
4. Fluid replacement is important. Fill your boda bag with water instead of brandy. Slightly warm water is fine; it shouldn't be too cold. Water is best but juice or herbal tea is okay too. Coffee, colas, and alcohol are dehydrating.

## SARAJEVO '84
### 5,000-Calorie Diet

| Sources of Carbohydrate | For 55 percent | For 65 percent |
|---|---|---|
| **Breakfast** | | |
| milk, lowfat | 2 cups | 1 cup |
| orange juice | ½ cup | 1½ cups |
| strawberries | ¾ cup | ¾ cup |
| soft-boiled eggs | 2 | 2 |
| fried sliced bacon | 2 slices | |
| porridge | 1½ cups | 1½ cups |
| raisin bread | 2 slices | 2 slices |
| butter | 2 tsps. | 2 tsps. |
| **Snack** | | |
| pear | 1 small | 1 small |
| red grapes | 12 | 24 |
| Shaklee fruit bar | | 1 |
| **Snack** | | |
| cheese | 2 oz. | 2 oz. |
| roll | 1 | 1 |
| green grapes | | 24 |
| **Lunch** | | |
| milk (low-fat) | 1 cup | 1 cup |
| vegetable soup | 1½ cups | 1½ cups |
| grilled strip steak | 3 oz. | 3 oz. |
| boiled potatoes | 1½ cups | 1½ cups |
| boiled beet leaves | 1 cup | 1 cup |
| cabbage sauté | ½ cup | ½ cup |
| kidney bean salad | | |
| rolls | | 2 |
| butter | 3 tsps. (1 tbsps.) | |
| apple | 1 small | 1 small |

| Sources of Carbohydrate | For 55 percent | For 65 percent |
|---|---|---|
| **Snack** | | |
| raisins | 4 tbsps. | 4 tbsps. |
| orange | 1 small | 1 small |
| banana | 1 small | 1 small |
| bread | | 1 slice |
| **Snack** | | |
| black bread | 4 slices | 4 slices |
| jam | 4 tbsps. | 4 tbsps. |
| butter | 2 tsps. | |
| Shaklee fruit bar | | |
| **Dinner** | | |
| milk (low-fat) | 1 cup | 1 cup |
| grilled mackerel | 3 oz. | 3 oz. |
| saffron rice | 2 cups | 2 cups |
| pasta | 2½ cups | 2½ cups |
| with tomato sauce | 1½ cups | 1½ cups |
| Brussels sprouts | 1 cup | 1 cup |
| cut wax beans | ½ cup | ½ cup |
| butter | 3 tsps. (1tbsp.) | |
| ice cream | ½ cup | 1 cup |
| **Snack** | | |
| milk (low-fat) | 1 cup | 1 cup |
| whole wheat bread | 2 slices | 2 slices |
| butter | 1 tsp. | |
| honey | 1 tbsp. | 1 tbsp. |
| fresh tomatoes with | 1 cup | 1 cup |
| dressing | 3 tbsps. | 2 tbsps. |
| fruit salad | 1 cup | 1 cup |

# CHAPTER ELEVEN

# Boxing

No other sport has had as many ups and downs over the years as boxing. Age-old, befitting an athletic form that is a straight outgrowth of primitive fighting, fisticuffs has traversed the millennia from sport to gladiatorial combat to banishment (for over a thousand years) and back to glory in nineteenth-century England. Since then it has seen heights of great pugilists like John L. Sullivan, Gentleman Jim Corbett, Ruby Robert Fitzsimmons ("the bigger they come, the harder they fall"), Jack Johnson and Jack Dempsey, Rocky Graziano and Rocky Marciano, Sugar Ray Robinson and Sugar Ray Leonard, and probably the two greatest—Joe Louis and Muhammad Ali. But it has also witnessed the lows of the houndings of the same Jack Johnson and Muhammad Ali, as well as huge fluctuations in popularity. The peaks came in the Golden Age of Dempsey, Tunney, and others, in the 1920's, the super-saturation of infant television in the early 1950's, and the excitement of everything Ali did from his second defeat of Sonny Liston in Lewiston, Maine, onward, especially whenever Smokin' Joe Frazier got into the same ring. The valleys included the doldrums of the 1930's, Joe Louis's Bum of the Month Club tour, the down days during World War II, and the most dramatic plunge of all, the fall from grace in the mid-1950's from a combination of overexposure, lack of interesting personalities in the ring, and too many interesting personalities involved outside of it.

Boxing has survived all of the reports of its death, though, and all of its doomsayers, because it is, along with running, ultimately a natural activity. Moreover, it is the quintessential male sport. As legalized hand-to-hand warfare, it allows the direct and vicarious (for the spectators) venting of the atavistic drives to defeat the enemy in open and fair combat. It's knightly jousting for Everyman. A sport where guts and ambition can carry a neophyte a long way (Tennessee Williams's "I coulda' been a contenda' " is almost as sanguine and certainly much more realistic a boast than "I could have been the Heavyweight Champion of the World"), it is also a sport where conditioning is as paramount a concern as combinations. The grueling matches, even though they no longer go beyond fifteen rounds as they did in the old days—John L. Sullivan once took *seventy-five* rounds in the sweltering heat of a Mississippi summer to bludgeon, bare fisted, his valiant opponent into submission—still require awesome stamina if one is getting beaten upon the whole time. Running out of gas before it's over is as costly to a boxer as a race car driver. Perhaps the most memorable example is Muhammad Ali's conquest over a considerably bigger, younger, and stronger then-World Champion George Foreman. Using a tactic called the "rope-a-dope," Ali turned himself into a human punching bag against the strangely loose ropes until big George wilted from the exertion in Kinshasa, Zaire's heat and humidity.

Training, roadwork, and the like obviously play a critical role in a boxer's preparations for a fight. But nutrition is certainly not ignored. Making weight, of course, is the most visible aspect of diet control. If a fighter is shooting for the junior welterweight crown, for example, he must weigh in—not fight —at or below 140 pounds. There is no margin for error. You can lose a shot at the title (the fight could go on but wouldn't count as a sanctioned junior welterweight bout) or forfeit a crown for as little as a half a pound excess avoirdupois. There is one exception, however. While the rule applies from flyweight (not over 112 pounds) through light heavyweight (not over 175 pounds), there is no limit on the big boys, the heavyweights. From "Two-Ton" Tony Galento to three-hundred-pound Buster Mathis (and Ed "Too Tall" Jones), the ring has witnessed some large individuals. And usually they couldn't beat the smaller but more talented and quicker guys. Witness what Max Baer did to the mammoth Primo Carnera in order to take the heavyweight crown, although, at a not insubstantial 210 pounds, he was still outweighed by forty-five pounds. Incidentally, Carnera was one of the first fighters to advertise his diet. According to his manager's press release, his daily breakfast consisted of a quart of orange juice, two quarts of milk, nineteen pieces of toast, fourteen eggs, a loaf of bread, and half a pound of Virginia ham. Just one in a long line of fistic hyperboles.

The following, however, is the real thing, from some great fighters and managers.

By his own admission the greatest boxer ever, **Muhammad Ali** is different from every other fighter who has made the same boast—he just might be right. The only man to have won the Heavyweight title three times, almost impossible to hit while in his prime, Ali still had the punching power to post thirty-seven of his fifty-six wins (out of sixty-one bouts) by knockouts. Born Cassius Marcellus Clay in Louisville, Kentucky, he won a Gold Medal in the 1960 Olympics as a light heavyweight. From then on it was on to bigger and better, doing his most damage in the 210–212 pound range. The rest truly is boxing history.

During his heyday as a fighter Ali was known to eat well. He even traveled with his own cook. In fact, when Ali did have trouble in the latter part of his career, it was often due to his weight increasing as a result of his great love of food. He was constantly forced to cut down in order to be able to fight at his best weight. He was also devoted to vitamins and these two liquid lubrications:

1. A drink devised for Ali by Dick Gregory, called 'Champ Juice' which both gives energy and flushes the system. Extract and strain the juice from eight lemons, four oranges, one grapefruit, and one lime, then combine them in a one gallon bottle. Stir in two cups of pure maple syrup, fill the bottle with distilled water, and keep in the refrigerator.
2. This one is a pure energy giver. In a blender, put two

avocados minus the skin and seed, a small onion, three garlic cloves, the juice from two lemons, and a quarter cup each of olive oil and honey. Fill the rest of the jar with V-8 juice before blending.

Nowadays his tastes are slightly more conventional, but he still has to keep his weight under control. His diet is well planned, giving him energy and helping him with his weight. For breakfast he has eggs straight up or cold cereal and milk with fruit slices on top, plus a slice of whole grain toast (no butter), a glass of milk, and a glass of fresh orange juice. Lunch is simply a green salad to which he adds tuna fish. Dinner is either beef, or his preference, chicken or fish, baked or broiled (never fried), with broccoli or green beans. His only weakness is desserts, which are the only things he can't duck.

**Smokin' Joe Frazier** is the man universally identified as Ali's chief opponent, winning one out of three. Winner of the Olympic Gold Medal in the Heavyweight Division in 1964, Frazier became the undisputed Heavyweight Champion of the World when he beat Ali in 1971. Now the boxing focus is on his son Marvis, who recently completed an unusual double, defeating English heavyweight Joe Bugner, ten years after his father performed the same feat. In fact, the Frazier family is a veritable conglomerate of fighters. Besides Marvis there is Frazier's other son, Hector, who fights as "Smokin' Joe Junior" plus two nephews, Rodney and Mark.

No one can say that Frazier doesn't take care of his boys. In fact, once a week he can be caught whipping up a gallon of a special brew called Smokey's Remedy that he claims gives energy, cures all ailments, and just might be the reason (along with talent) for the great success of all the Fraziers. Unfortunately we will have to wait until all of their fighting days are over before he will reveal his secret recipe. Suffice it to say that the secret brew has been described as being of a brownish color with some kind of oil base, that it smells of mint, and there are whole pieces of fruit mixed in. Frazier gives it to his boys every morning before breakfast.

After the drink, Joe will have four eggs plus bacon, sausage, and grits along with two glasses of fresh orange juice. Breakfast for Marvis will be three scrambled eggs plus bacon and sausages. Lunch for Joe when he has it, which isn't all the time, consists of a sandwich, usually steak or cheese, with some fruit punch but no dessert. Lunch for Marvis, on the other hand, is another Frazier concoction. This is a high protein mixture (another secret) that contains milk powder, but this one has no fruit to make it taste good. In fact, Joe admits that it tastes awful. I guess it builds discipline as well as stamina. Dinner for both father and son is generally the same. They love porterhouse steaks along with baked potatoes with butter. They always have leafy green vegetables (greens of all kinds are a big part of their diet), a salad, and a couple of large glasses of fruit juice, orange mixed with cranberry being their favorite.

Joe's general dietary rules for all the Fraziers are to be careful about what they eat. They like meat, but eat a great deal of fish as well. They never use salt and eat plenty of vegetables. For snacks they eat oranges and suck on lemons. Candy bars, cookies, and junk food are not in the Frazier household corner.

**Larry Holmes** is the man who replaced Ali as the world's premier heavyweight, and who has rather easily disposed of all challenges to his title since he took it in 1978. Holmes is a believer in listening to what his body tells him. Certainly there is no one around who will argue with him.

Holmes finds that he does his best fighting at 215 pounds. To stay at that weight, he echoes the practice of a lot of the big men in football; he eats only two meals a day. To combine these two ideas, if he feels a desire for something he usually doesn't eat, like a Danish, he will substitute it for his usual breakfast, not add it on. Breakfast is normally three eggs (over easy) with ham, English muffins (without butter but sometimes with jelly), and coffee. For dinner, his big meal, Holmes likes red meat (New York strip steaks) or fish plus "all kinds of fresh vegetables, my favorites being corn, broccoli, and rice." Every once in a while during training he will have some fried chicken as a treat, but overall he is very careful about what he eats. Holmes's advice to everyone is "to definitely avoid junk foods. Occasionally a hot dog is okay, but a good diet is extremely important to a fighter." One element for that diet could be the following dish specially whipped up for Holmes by the Dunes Hotel in Las Vegas; Larry Holmes Trout. A simple recipe to prepare, it consists of a fresh boned trout put on tin foil, marinated with salt, pepper, and lemon juice, and browned. After it is cooked the skin is removed.

**Marvelous Marvin Hagler** is considered by many of boxing's experts to be, pound for pound, the best boxer around today. That's because he has it all—speed of hand and foot, power in both hands, ability to take a tough shot, stamina, and mental toughness. The Middleweight Champion of the World since 1980, Hagler has lost only two bouts in his entire professional career. Hagler is one of the only fighters to be a consensus world champion, holding down both the World Boxing Council and the World Boxing Association Middleweight Titles. While only a handful would want to take him on in the ring, a little known fact is that few would want to parry with him in the kitchen either. "I have a dynamite recipe for meatloaf," he confesses, "and I especially enjoy cooking an early morning exotic breakfast." Something one wouldn't normally associate with a man who had forty-seven knockouts in sixty fights.

Nutrition, in fact, is an important part of his training. "Ever since I started boxing I have maintained essentially the same nutritional program. I am my own specialist because I know what is best for me. Fighters are different from other athletes. You know, different strokes for different folks." And Marvelous Marvin knows them all. In training, he relies on fish, salad, and a vegetable. Following the weigh in on the day of the fight, however, he will eat red meat and plenty of spaghetti.

Hagler can also be classified as sensible. He regularly takes B complex, C, E, and "pregnancy pill" (minerals and iron) supplements, and between bouts he eats "a little bit of everything —but in moderation." His special high energy drink is simply orange juice with added extra vitamin C. His philosophy for youngsters is thoughtful as well: "Avoid cigarettes, alcohol, and drugs of any kind. Love and honor your mother and father and heed their advice on what is good for you because they know more than you do and can give you proper guidance." Pretty marvelous stuff, all right.

**Tyrell Biggs,** the six foot, five inch superheavyweight contender, is the U.S. hope among the big men in this year's Olympics. Biggs hopes to emulate some of the other great professional careers of U.S. Olympians, and has already followed in their dietary footsteps.

"I stay away from junk and I drink no alcohol. To maintain my weight I eat a lot, but it's a lot of the right foods. I used to eat everything, but now that I watch what I eat I find that I feel better and I box better as well." Breakfast for Biggs will be large, since like Holmes, he doesn't eat again until dinner. He'll have orange juice plus three eggs, bacon or a large bowl of cereal, oatmeal or cream of wheat. While he's training he has no lunch, just some fruit, oranges, apples, and bananas. Dinner will be substantial. "I don't eat pork, but like steak, hamburgers, chicken, or fish along with two vegetables, usually spinach, string beans, or peas, along with a baked potato, and occasionally a salad. "Two days before a match, I'll cut out the salads as too much roughage might upset my stomach. I eat no dessert except fresh fruit, never pies or cakes, although occasionally I will have some ice cream. And while I'm normally not into vitamin supplements, if I'm tired on a particular day I'll take a $B_{12}$ tablet for energy."

**Roosevelt Sanders, Jr.,** coach of the U.S. Men's Olympic Boxing Team and the national cordinator of the Amateur Boxing Federation, approves of Biggs's diet as he feels that proper nutrition is important. "What we take in has a direct bearing on how we are going to perform. The important thing for fighters to remember is not just to start seven days before a competition to get into shape but to start a month or more ahead of time. Some young fighters wait until a day or two before the fight to get in shape and they are just killing themselves." Here is Coach Sanders' preparation program for a bout:

"A month before the competition start eating (if you don't always) a well-balanced diet including meat, chicken, fish, fowl, and vegetables. Do not bulk up on any one category. Carbohydrate loading for a boxer is not good. Bulky food tends to slow down a boxer. Here we look for speed and agility.

"An ideal breakfast would be one or two eggs (a heavyweight should have three) along with a slice of toast and a glass of juice,

230

orange being the best. I highly recommend hot tea with lemon as a drink. Use only honey as a sweetener and avoid milk which tends to sour in the stomach.

"For lunch I generally recommend a salad (while in training camp, however, the boxers only eat fruit). A small amount of cheese and tuna fish or other high protein food is also good. I don't recommend meat, though, as it is too heavy at this time. The drink again should be hot tea and lemon which is a favorite of most professional boxers.

"Dinner ideally should be poultry or fish, lean meats, a salad, and vegetables along with a slice of bread. Ice cream is okay for dessert if they want something sweet. If they are hungry during the day and at night I always recommend snacking on fresh fruit —oranges, apples, pears, plums, or cantaloupe.

"When the fight is at seven-thirty this is my recommendation for a good prefight meal. At two or three o'clock in the afternoon have a small portion of fish or poultry, green leafy vegetables such as spinach, plus a small portion of ice cream and peaches which are both light but filling. Tea is also good here as it tends to stimulate the body. The object of the prefight meal is to fill the body up but by the time the boxer is ready to fight, all the food has been digested. The body and reflexes are faster, and there is nothing to slow him down. In the days of Joe Louis everyone believed that a big steak before a fight was the thing to have. Now we believe in a balanced meal that has light proteins. If athletes need quick energy, they should eat a candy bar, but remember, plain chocolate, no nuts or fillings which could cause an upset stomach."

Ali's trainer, and the trainer of eight other world champions, was **Angelo Dundee,** one of boxing's living legends. Dundee's other title holders are: Sugar Ray Leonard (welterweight), Jimmy Ellis (heavyweight), Willy Pastrano (light heavyweight), Carmen Basilio (welterweight and middleweight), Ralph Dupas (junior middleweight), Jose Napoles (another welterweight), Sugar Ramos (featherweight), and Luis Rodriguez (yet another welterweight).

Dundee feels that a young fighter's system will burn up practically anything he puts into it. However his recommendation for them is to eat sensibly and to choose foods that agree with them. "Sugar Ray Leonard, for example, was not a big eater. He never ate too much at one sitting. However he likes cheeseburgers and they agreed with him, so before each fight he ate a cheeseburger."

Actually Dundee prefers his fighters to eat a high protein diet of fish, chicken, and steak. If they want to lose weight, all they have to do is to cut down on the intake. He insists that his men avoid all drugs and alcohol. He also believes that young athletes have an inbred natural selection process and should listen to their bodies and find out what works for and against them. For everything else, though, they should listen to the trainer.

**Jackie McCoy** is another superstar trainer, having trained many world champions—including Don Jordan (welterweight), Raul Rojas (featherweight), Mando Ramos (lightweight), Rodolfo Gonzalez (another lightweight) and, most recently, welterweight champion Carlos Palomino.

McCoy also believes it is a fallacy that boxers need a lot of meat before a fight. "Carbohydrates like spaghetti and pancakes are an important prefight meal, along with conventional things like steak, salad, and vegetables. Fighters have what we call a dry out; they eat at three the day before a fight and then fast until they weigh in at noon the next day. They take off up to two pounds by doing this alone in order to make weight, but then they have to eat again to build up strength for the fight that evening. Some of the fighters have their own special methods to build up for a fight. Carlos Palomino, for example, is Mexican, but before a fight he avoids his favorite foods, which are starches, tacos, enchiladas, etc., and eats a high protein diet with some vegetables. My advice is to use good common sense."

**Jimmy Jacobs** is the manager for many world class fighters, including Edwin Rosario, the world lightweight champion, and Wilfred Benitez, one of the very few boxers to hold three different world championships—junior welterweight, welterweight, and junior middleweight. Jacobs feels that trying to come up with an ideal diet for all his fighters "would be like Ann Landers trying to give the same solution for everyone's marital problems. The individual fighters and their situations are so different. The most important thing for a fighter to be is psychologically fit; he has to believe in what he is doing. If he believes, for example, that eating eight oranges a day will help make him a better fighter, it usually does. Rosario, on the other hand, eats like he's going to the electric chair. In training for his championship fights he would eat three cheeseburgers with french fries and then proceed to burn it all off, but Benitez would cut out everything, even water, when he was trying to get down to his desired weight." As said, different strokes for different folks.

**Cus D'Amato** is another legendary trainer of champions, like Floyd Patterson. D'Amato feels that fighters really have only six or seven peak years and they have to make the most of them. "I believe that high protein and low carbohydrates work better for most fighters. Steaks, lamb chops, and chicken along with salads are good methods to reduce and maintain an ideal weight. Green vegetables are also important for fighters.

"Boxers as a whole have to be disciplined. If a man has to make a hundred-sixty-pound contract, he has to exercise that discipline. Some fighters stop drinking liquids two days before the fight (drying out). Then they also have to be strict; they can't even have water. In my opinion, and I have been around all the old-timers, few things have changed. There is and always will be a psychological factor to boxing. Many boxers believe that certain things are detrimental—you can't have coffee and you can't smoke. They do drink tea, but avoid things like fried foods. They even say sex on the night before a fight is bad, and most fighters believe this as well.

"A boxer's diet should be as follows: For breakfast he should have eggs, toast, and hot tea. He should only have milk or juice if he doesn't have to worry about his weight. My light heavyweight champ Jose Torres, for example, had to cut out all orange juice to lose weight. Breakfast should be eaten after the morning run. He then trains until one or two o'clock and that's when he should have his big meal: steaks and lamb chops, chicken along with green vegetables, a salad, and a few slices of toast. On this diet a boxer will never have to worry about weight. Charley Phil Rosenberg, the great bantamweight champion back in the

1920's, went from one hundred sixty-five pounds to one hundred eighteen pounds on this diet."

In words that have stirred generations of great boxers, D'Amato explained his overall philosophy: "As I mentioned before, a fighter must have his mind mentally in tune as well as his diet. He must think winning is possible, and if not, he will fail. As far as energy goes, that's a different story. Some people compare boxing to street fighting, the Rocky Graziano types. But in street fights there is anger and in boxing in the ring the fighter is not angry at anyone. The adrenaline that he pumps brings constant fear and fear is his best friend. Nature gave us fear in order to survive, but it can be like a snowball and unless you keep it under control it can destroy you. It all boils down to a matter of discipline for both the body and mind. When the boxer steps into the ring he cannot let the fear in his mind exaggerate when he faces his opponent. He must learn to live with this fear in order to become two people; the mind and body separate and the mind can then direct the body. In a professional boxer this is achieving Zen, the mind is impersonal, it is detached.

"The philosphy of the trainer is to make the boxer feel that he's the best but not to let him test it until he knows he can beat the best. And all this takes is discipline in every area. Diet is one of the areas, and if one does well there he will do the same mentally as well."

**Dave Gorman,** who counts among his boxers Welterweight Champion of the World, Donald Curry, feels that the boxers are under such a strict training program during the season that when they have some time off they really "hog" it up. "That's okay, but man, they *really* suffer when they go back into training. Breakfast during training should be light: freshly squeezed juices or maybe a grapefruit or an orange. Lunch should be the main meal, as eating later in the day the fighter just goes to sleep on a full stomach and those calories turn to fat. At lunch the boxer will have a steak, with a baked potato, salad, and fresh vegetables with some spaghetti on the side for added carbohydrates. The core of the lunch, though, should be vegetables and good beef. Dessert is nothing, as most of the fighters are watching their weight. But if they must have something sweet they should have it now instead of later in the evening. Dinner is just soup, like chicken noodle or vegetable, something light and easily digestible."

For the prefight meal, Gorman's program is slightly different. "The weigh-in is at noon and then the boxer does not go into the ring until eight o'clock at night. Lunch then would be a small portion of red meat and a small portion of spaghetti. Later in the afternoon, about two hours before the event, he can then have a small piece of fish, an excellent source of high protein that is low in fat, along with a bowl of soup, nothing heavy. I suggest they don't have meat within eight hours of competition as it tends to make them sluggish. **Donald Curry,** who follows this program, has really learned to take care of himself. "When I first met him" says Gorman, "he had pancakes loaded with maple syrup for breakfast. That might be good for other sports, but for boxing it is just too much food."

Gorman's wife, Loretta, works with his boxers in planning their vitamin regime and this is what she suggests: "Boxers should take a thousand milligrams of vitamin E daily, along with a thousand milligrams of C and a good multiple vitamin with a high B content. I give them B complex as well, but in a series of four days on, four days off, as we have found that they get sluggish if they take it all the time. Five days before a fight I put them on potassium. This is good as the fighter sweats a lot and loses this valuable mineral. I also cut out the multiple vitamin and B's at this time and keep them on C and E. If a person takes vitamins daily, a few days off of them won't hurt and I've found that if you don't eat (for fighters drying out) the B tends to make you nauseous and the multiple vitamin increases the appetite. I've also discovered riboflavin is good for fighters that bruise a lot and iron tablets can counteract the weakness that comes from loss of blood."

# CHAPTER TWELVE

# Running

To most of us, even those who recreationally jog the odd mile or two per day, running is a straightforward affair. Right, left, right, left. But for the experts, the athletes and coaches engaged in track events, it is much more complex than that. Starting block posture, stride, gait, leg lift, arm motions, and body lean are all studied in the most minute detail to shave tenths-of-seconds off times.

That is just for running on a straightaway. Add curves and you have a whole new set of forces and vectors to contend with. Then you can really get complicated—litter the path with left-over pieces of a picket fence, and just for fun call them hurdles. Now one has to figure out running and jumping without breaking stride or losing momentum. Let's not even think about events like the triple jump or steeplechase.

So much for the idea that running is a simple sport. It requires as much discipline and concentration as any other at the world-class level. To blaze at high speed requires a body that is pure machine. And keeping up a killing pace for five thousand or ten thousand meters, or a marathon, demands the right fuel. It's not surprising that the top runners are among those athletes most interested in diet ideas and their advisers among the best informed.

The world's preeminent middle distance runner has to be Oregon's **Mary Decker,** the current world champion in both the fifteen hundred and three thousand meters. A superbly versatile superstar, Decker holds world records in the eight hundred meter, the one thousand meter, the fifteen hundred meter, the mile, the five thousand meter, and the ten thousand meter. She is also the winner of the 1982 USA/Mobil Grand Prix, conducted by The Athletics Congress, and the Jean Naté Grand Prix. Besides being one of our leading Olympic hopefuls, Decker is also a media darling because of her dramatic personal life, comprising numerous medical marvels and a troubled marriage to Ron Tabb, a top marathoner.

While it is most unlikely that it was a cause of their marital strains, Decker did confide that she used to eat better before she was married. "Ron eats more junk than I do." Decker believes in eating a balanced diet for energy, including proteins, vegetables, and carbohydrates. She also believes in the theory of eating only when hungry. "I try to eat carbohydrates at least three or four hours before I run. In the morning, hot cereal is a good source, and throughout the day foods such as bread, baked potatoes, and spaghetti are easy to digest and energy-giving."

As a middle to long distance runner, Decker must be concerned with stamina. Her advice: "Contrary to some opinion, sugar does not give sustaining energy for runners. It simply gives you a high for a while and then drops you to a low that was worse than before. When you are extremely tired, it is best to cut back a little bit on your mileage when you train, rather than push yourself. However, eating well plus taking vitamins (in my case, B complex, C, and E) will give you more sustaining strength and keep you healthy."

It was a full twenty years ago that an American female runner last caught the public's fancy as has Decker. That woman was **Wilma Rudolph,** who won three gold medals as a sprinter in the 1964 Olympics in Tokyo. Today, Rudolph, a mother of four and an Olympic supporter as a spokesperson for Minute Maid juices, stays trim and healthy with plenty of exercise and "a well-balanced diet." Among her favorite foods are macaroni with broccoli and other simple foods. An example of her sprinter's philosophy of keeping it light but with plenty of power is her "Protein Punch Smoothie," a blend of crushed walnuts, half a banana, orange juice, and an egg. "It's nutritious, healthful, and delicious."

Another maternal runner is **Chie Matsuda,** Japan's top woman marathoner. Mother of two, Matsuda balances her homelife with that of a star athlete as well as her work for the Sheisado cosmetic firm.

Nutrition is an important subject for Matsuda. "I generally like to run before breakfast and then eat a very large meal consisting of vegetables, a protein like meat or fish plus rice, and bread. Lunch is the same, only smaller portions, and dinner is the same as well but with more vegetables such as cabbage and tomatoes. A good dinner is beef boiled with fresh vegetables and served over rice (no soy sauce, however—too much salt). I also drink milk three times a day for calcium.

"A very popular Japanese dish is made with tofu, which is very high in protein. The meal is a high energy giver: Chop assorted vegetables in a pan, add tofu, chicken, and consommé that you can buy in an Oriental market. Add a tablespoon of sake and a tablespoon of soy sauce and boil for twenty minutes. Dessert is fresh fruit."

Matsuda finds that a high energy snack is the Japanese delicacy sushi, known affectionately to most of us as raw fish. This is a classic case of going with foods that you are used to and with which your body is familiar. Few Western athletes would feel comfortable with such a lean pure protein "snack." On the other hand, Matsuda also believes in eating heavy protein and vegetables a week before a race and adding carbohydrates just three days before. Sports are international, diet consciousness is too, but what you eat doesn't always translate as easily as yards into meters.

Local habits and tolerances are exhibited by another runner from Matsuda's side of the globe, New Zealander **Rod Dixon** winner of the 1983 New York Marathon. Known as having one of the longest, most successful and varied racing careers, Dixon in one stretch won sixteen of his twenty road races in 1981 (setting course records in Philadelphia, Lynchburg, and Maggie Valley). Among the top distance runners in the world throughout the 1980's, Dixon's concession to being in his 30's has been to lengthen his races. Three times a New Zealand Olympian, he was a bronze medalist in the fifteen hundred meter in 1972 in Munich. Now he runs a mile just to warm up.

Dixon's basic diet is lots of fresh vegetables and plenty of fiber. He also likes pizza and hamburgers, but what sets him apart is the amazing amount of beer he drinks—about two or three pints a day. Someone once said that Dixon never met a beer he didn't like. But like native Bavarian soccer great Franz Beckenbauer, Dixon's Down Under background prepared him to handle the stuff. Otherwise, his diet is exemplary. Breakfast is usually a bran cereal and a bran muffin, while lunch before training is light and consists of fresh fruit or steamed vegetables. Dinner is meat or fish, vegetables, and a dessert such as ice cream. And, of course, beer.

**Doug Brown** is also a three-time Olympian, having been on the U.S. Olympic Team in 1972, 1976, and 1980. A five-time National Champion, he is an American record-holder in the 3,000 meter steeplechase.

Brown, like Decker, runs under the auspices of Athletics West, a full service club financed by Nike. The same age as Dixon, Brown is another runner who defies the prevalent view of an athlete's prime: "It's hard to believe, but at thirty-one, a runner is considered old. Most of the champions are in their early twenties, and done by the time they are thirty. I think, however, if you're in good shape and take care of yourself, there is no such thing as being too old for anything."

Brown feels that one way to stay in great shape is to watch your diet. "You don't have to be fanatic about it, but make sure it's well-rounded. A good tip for runners is to always eat after you've run, not before. You shouldn't have much in your stomach up to three hours before you start."

After running for five or six miles in the morning, Brown has a protein-rich breakfast of eggs, bacon, toast, and milk. Breakfast is the only meal at which he has a high concentration of proteins; the rest of the day he eats more carbohydrates, adding quiche, spaghetti, and bread to his balanced meals. Two days before a competition he goes even heavier on the carbohydrates and feels that something like pizza is a good food for this.

As for vitamins, "If you're eating properly you probably don't need them, but just to make sure you cover any deficiency (even a one percent deficiency can make a difference in a top athlete) it is a good idea to take them just to hedge your bets." His program includes a liver pill for iron, vitamin B complex, a time-released C, a multiple vitamin, and a multi-mineral supplement.

"Common sense is important in nutrition. Most runners need three good meals a day. There is no miracle energy pill, but I might have three or four cups of coffee about two hours before a big race to feel good and jittery." Being familiar with Dixon's liquid diet, I asked Brown if in addition to pumping caffeine into an empty prerace stomach, he indulged in other unorthodox refreshments, like alcohol. "Only to excess!" he replied. But he feels there is a mitigating factor, if not justification. "When you're in great shape you hardly ever get hangovers. The heart is a muscle, and when you're fit, it can pump much more blood than when you're out of shape. Therefore, the alcohol gets out of your system quicker." Well, at least no one has ever been recklessly hurdled by a besotted steeplechaser.

**Bill Rodgers** of Boston is probably the single best known marathoner in the U.S. The King of the Roads, Rodgers is a four-time Boston and four-time New York Marathon champion, a former American record holder in the marathon, and world record holder over thirty thousand meters. The Wayne Gretzky of runners, Rodgers eats both frequently and in quantity. He'll wake up at four o'clock in the morning just to eat. He likes "junk" food such as pizza, ice cream, and potato chips, and his specialty is eating mayonnaise by the spoonful, at any hour.

Rodgers usually eats about five meals a day. When he gets up in the morning he has a bran muffin and juice, then goes out for his morning run. Upon his return he will have a salad and some cranberry bread. Cheese in the afternoon bridges lunchtime, with his big meal being in the evening. For dinner he is big on all kinds of seafood (lobster Newburg is a favorite), but doesn't eat too much red meat.

Basically, his diet is one of complex carbohydrates and fiber although he does not load carbohydrates. The day before a race, however, he cuts out all the junk food to cleanse his system. Probably his favorite meal would be fish and mayonnaise—and an extra roll.

**Bill Fink** works at the Human Performance Laboratory at Ball State University in Muncie, Indiana, and is one of the pioneers in this country of sports-related biophysical research. The lab, run by the legendary Dr. David Costill, studies exercise physiology, muscle metabolism, and nutrition. In fact, it is the largest lab of its kind, and one of the first to do extensive testing on athletes and measure "muscle make-up." Muscles are made up of "slow twitches" and "fast twitches." If you have a high percentage of fast twitch you are said to most likely be more successful as a sprinter, with slow twitch, a marathoner. Rodgers, for example, has a 70 percent slow twitch, so he is clearly going with his strength in the marathon. They were also among the first to test oxygen intake (lung capacity) on a treadmill and break down the body into a stick figure on a computer to show how you have to change your form to make it more efficient. In general, biophysical research was initially the sole province of the East Germans, but Ball State brought it to America.

The following diet for runners was recommended by Fink: "First of all, runners in general tend to be light weight people, and if you're not burning up two thousand calories a day it is advisable not to eat extremely large portions.

## The Runner's Diet

*Breakfast:* Rather than bacon or eggs, the breakfast of a runner should be high in carbohydrates. Pancakes, waffles, cold cereals, toast, and an orange or other fruit juices are a good start. Coffee, if desired as a beverage can be had, but not because caffeine does anything for you.

*Lunch* on the run, so to speak, should also be carbohydrates, although it is difficult to have a complete carbohydrate sandwich. You have to put something inside the bread. Be sure to have two slices or more of bread, however, with fruit for dessert or a fruit yogurt.

*Dinner,* or a sit down lunch, would include variety for well-rounded nutrition. Italian pasta with bread is good for the carbohydrates. Chinese food is excellent—try a large helping or two of rice with sprouts on it. Or the standard American meat-and-potatoes dinner is fine, but go heavy on the potatoes. Vegetables and salad are also good carbohydrates but they are not particularly high in calories, and when we talk about carbohydrates we speak of carbohydrates for calories and that means the heavier ones, the breads, etc. So have them along with vegetables. Avoid fatty foods, mainly because they hang around in the stomach for a long time and cause a feeling of indigestion and discomfort.

*Snacks* in between can include liquids, soft drinks to replace carbohydrates, or yogurts and fruit, even milk and cookies.

The classic regime of carbohydrate loading that was popular a few years ago is generally not recommended by Fink. "The runners ate all fat and protein (a bit like the old Stillman diet) for three days early in the week, thereby depleting all their carbohydrates. Then for the remaining three days prior to a race, they would eat just carbohydrates. The problem is that the early part of this regime can make someone hypoglycemic and terribly irritable. It is wise simply to add more carbohydrates in the form of bread, pasta, rice, etc. without cutting back to begin with. The secret is to exercise more than you eat. The body needs the exercise stimulus to store more carbohydrates. What we call a depletion bout—burning off glycogen—is stimulus for the body to store more. If you eat too much protein or fat, however, it won't deplete. You have to burn it off. I always say you have to *work for your food.* When the glycogen is burned off, it stimulates the enzymes to produce more. If the muscles are already full of glycogen, the carbohydrates will simply be converted to fat."

Fink's advice for the weekend athlete looking to lose weight is equally intriguing: "Many people feel that by eating a high protein diet they will automatically become thinner and therefore have more energy to run. This is, however, false. The program works by emptying the body of carbohydrates, that's all. It's like taking all the gas out of a car's tank. The car will be lighter, naturally, but it will also have no fuel. Carbohydrates are your body's fuel. As you lose fuel your body becomes dehydrated as well, so between the water loss and the carbohydrate loss, people think they are losing weight. It is very deceptive. The minute you start eating normally again everything comes right back on. You have to be on what we call a negative caloric balance. Eat less food, cut out fat and decrease the protein, but keep eating some carbohydrates and you'll lose weight and have an incredible amount of energy. Also, when you eat carbohydrates you become less hungry.

"But before you even think about carbohydrate loading or simply eating a lot of carbohydrates you have to be doing something that requires more than an hour of physical activity.

"There is also a fallacy in thinking that eating something right before the sport will give you instant energy. For all runners and other athletes the axiom should be: 'Exercise today on what you ate yesterday, eat today for tomorrow.' We exercise on the carbohydrates already stored in the muscles. In fact, if you do eat something sugary before an exercise bout, there is a chance that you will become more tired. One of the effects of eating carbohydrates is that the pancreas puts out more insulin and then, when you begin to exercise, there is a precipitous drop in blood sugar.

"The best advice we can give to full-time and weekend runners is to eat a balanced diet, cut back on the fat and have a ration of fifty to sixty-five percent carbohydrates and twelve to fifteen percent protein."

**Dick Gregory** is a man of many trades. Besides his most well-known career as a social satirist and comedian, he has advised boxers, including Muhammad Ali, basketball players like Maurice Lucas, whole baseball teams (the White Sox) and runners. One of his most accomplished personal feats was running from Los Angeles to New York at a clip of fifty miles a day, every day for seventy-one days, all when he was forty-four years old. So he practices as well as preaches.

"The most important thing for a runner to remember is that his body is under constant stress. To counteract this he needs a proper diet and a great deal of rest. Most athletes do not get enough rest. The other thing to remember is that running is a very dehydrating sport (think of this—on a cold winter day if you're simply lying in bed you would use up as much as eight pints of liquid. You can imagine how much liquid you need if you do a sport such as running in July.)

"A good way to take liquids is to mix a tablespoon of honey into a gallon of distilled water with added lemon juice and drink this throughout the day. (See also his recipe for Champ Juice in the Boxing chapter.) I also feel that most of a runner's diet should be fruit. For example, a breakfast of ripe melons, grapes, oranges, pears (no apples as they can sometimes give stomach cramps), or ripe bananas would be excellent. Lunch should be a green salad with a dressing of olive oil, fresh lemon juice, and a little honey. Dinner is lightly steamed vegetables, a small salad, and forty minutes later some fruit. Nothing should be cooked. Grapes are a very important fruit as they are almost all liquid. Dried fruit, however, should only be eaten after soaking overnight. Otherwise it is too hard to digest. The day of the event, it is advisable to drink a lot of water and rest as much as three hours prior to the race and eat any amount of fruit.

"I also recommend the following vitamins to runners: Close to three thousand milligrams of time released vitamin C, a thousand units of A and five thousand of D, yeast tablets twice a day, four in the morning and four in the evening, along with a B complex, multi-vitamin, and multi-mineral, plus additional calcium, potassium, and magnesium. Bee pollen tablets also seem to help. I recommend one teaspoon of the granules or two tablets."

Finally, Gregory proposes the following vegetarian regime. As a counterpoint to all the diets prescribed for shedding pounds, and after hearing from all the athletes, coaches, and experts about all the various ideas for weight loss, it seems fitting to end this book with a classic health food fanatic's diet with a twist—how to gain weight.

*Dick Gregory's Vegetarian Gainer*

### Menu I

*Breakfast:*   tall glass of freshly squeezed grapefruit juice
old-fashioned rolled oats and dried prunes, figs, and/or apricots soaked in pure water overnight—

before serving, add a tablespoon of wheat germ and
sweeten with honey
glass of soy milk, seed milk, or nut milk

*Lunch:*  large salad of mixed vegetables—lettuce, celery,
carrots, radishes—topped with kelp, caraway seed,
sunflower seed, or sesame seed
lemonaise or a herb salad dressing may be used as
a topping

*Dinner:*  tall glass of fresh carrot or other vegetable juice
steamed turnip greens or spinach, squash, or beets
—sprinkle sesame seed or sunflower seed for topping
almonds or raisins may be used for dessert
cup of alfalfa or mint tea

## Menu II

*Breakfast:*  tall glass of freshly squeezed grapefruit juice
dish of berries in season, or fresh fruit sprinkled with
a tablespoon or two of wheat germ
cup of rosemary, peppermint, or anise tea

*Lunch:*  tall glass of fresh orange, tomato, or other fruit juice
soaked dried figs, prunes, and raisins mixed with ½
cup ground almonds, and a tablespoon of wheat
germ
glass of soy, seed, or nut milk

*Dinner:*  tall glass of fresh carrot or other vegetable juice
steamed string beans with flaked almonds
steamed shredded beets and carrots
cup of alfalfa or mint tea

## Menu III

*Breakfast:*  tall glass of fresh orange juice.
old-fashioned rolled oats soaked overnight
dried prunes, figs, and/or apricots soaked
overnight—

add 1 or 2 tablespoons of wheat germ and sweeten
with honey before serving
glass of soy, seed, or nut milk

*Lunch:*           tall glass of freshly squeezed grapefruit juice
large mixed vegetable salad—lettuce, carrots, cel-
ery—topped with sesame seed, sunflower seed, or
pumpkin seed, with lemonaise or other salad dressing
glass of soy, seed, or nut milk

*Dinner:*          tall glass of fresh carrot or other vegetable juice
cabbage salad: Shred equal parts red, white and
green cabbage and combine with finely chopped
carrot—add a teaspoon of dill seed and mix together
—top with pumpkin or sunflower seed and use lemonaise or a herb salad dressing to moisten
cup of alfalfa or mint tea

## Menu IV

*Breakfast:*     tall glass of freshly squeezed grapefruit juice
sliced fresh peaches or pears
4 ounces yogurt mixed with ¼ cup sunflower seeds
and ¼ cup finely ground pumpkin seeds and 1 tablespoon honey
cup of mint tea

*Lunch:*           tall glass of fresh carrot or other fresh vegetable
juice
a large tomato stuffed with yogurt and chopped nuts,
such as almonds, or seeds, sprinkled with wheat
germ
an apple for dessert
glass of soy, seed, or nut milk

*Dinner:*          tall glass of fresh vegetable juice
steamed cabbage topped with caraway seeds and/or
sunflower or sesame seeds

246

steamed beets and steamed cauliflower may be
served in combination
cup of alfalfa or mint tea

## Menu V

*Breakfast:*  tall glass of freshly squeezed orange or grapefruit
juice.
sliced bananas sprinkled with wheat germ—add a
tablespoon of honey and top with sprinkled almonds
glass of soy, seed, or nut milk

*Lunch:*  tall glass of fresh carrot or other freshly made vegetable juice
shredded cabbage and grated carrot salad, with
minced onion and minced parsley, topped with
lemonaise or a herb salad dressing—serve on romaine lettuce—pumpkin, sesame, and sunflower
seeds may also be added to taste
glass of soy, seed, or nut milk

*Dinner:*  glass of fresh vegetable juice
steamed asparagus, steamed beets, steamed okra,
topped with sunflower seeds or sesame seeds
cup of mint tea
later in the evening, some raisins and an apple

## Menu VI

*Breakfast:*  tall glass of freshly squeezed orange or grapefruit
juice
dish of peaches, berries in season or melon with 2
tablespoons wheat germ, 2 tablespoons ground almonds, 1 tablespoon honey
glass of soy, seed, or nut milk

*Lunch:*  tall glass of fresh carrot juice (or other fresh vegetable juice)
2 cups cubed apples, 1 cup raisins and 1 cup

chopped almonds mixed together with the juice of a lemon—add honey if desired
glass of soy, seed, or nut milk, or cup of herb tea

*Dinner:*  tall glass of fresh vegetable juice
mixed vegetable salad—lettuce, celery, parsley (chopped), and radishes—mixed with sesame seeds and topped with a herb salad dressing
steamed string beans, okra, and carrots if desired.
cup of alfalfa or mint tea

## Menu VII

*Breakfast:*  tall glass of freshly squeezed orange or grapefruit juice
If you have orange juice, then have ½ grapefruit topped with honey
old-fashioned rolled oats soaked overnight—add ground almonds, pecans or filberts, and 1 tablespoon wheat germ—mix well before serving
cup of rosemary, mint, or camomile tea

*Lunch:*  large tomato stuffed with yogurt and sprinkled with chopped nuts and wheat germ
glass of soy, seed, or nut milk

*Dinner:*  tall glass of fresh carrot or other vegetable juice
mix well: shredded cabbage, grated carrots, and chopped minced or grated onions, garnished with pumpkin, sunflower, or sesame seeds, and topped with a herb salad dressing
cup of mint, alfalfa, or other herbal tea

**Note:** "These sample menus are intended to give you an idea of the ingredients involved and possible combinations. I want to urge you, however, to be creative. Experiment with the items. Make your own favorites. I urge you not to mix fruits and vegetables together in the same meal. (There is a theory among strict vegetarians that you should not mix different food groups because the body can best handle one food group at a time.) Mixing fruit with vegetable juices, or vegetables with fruit juices, is all right. Be especially creative with seed garnishes. Get used to using sunflower seeds, sesame seeds, and pumpkin seeds. In salads, use them as you ordinarily would grated cheese or a hard-boiled egg.

"As an addition to the weight-on diet, use natural vitamin supplements, iron tablets, multi-vitamins, vitamin E, protein powder, tablet or liquid. You may take flaxseed before meals, and also brewers' yeast. Dried beans or peas may also be used. Get used to drinking herbal teas, peppermint, alfalfa, and the like, instead of coffee."

# Putting
# It Together

Wayne Gretzky feasts while Lawrence Taylor fasts. It would be easy to conclude that the length and breadth of the advice of the athletes and others revealed in the previous twelve chapters is so diverse as to have something for everyone and a rationalization for everything. But that analysis would be entirely wrong. What we've seen is a large number of superstars and super advisers advocating intelligent alternative nutritional concepts that can be adjusted according to each of our lifestyles and needs. The key is to find a blend that best suits your metabolism, build, and activity level.

While it would take another twelve chapters to restate the advice given by the experts, a few solid conclusions might be in order:

• Fresh is best. Stay away from highly processed foods and overcooked produce.
• Complex carbohydrates, especially whole grain breads, pasta, and potatoes, are much more desirable sources of energy than is sugar.
• Fiber should be an essential part of any diet. The right

amount, though, depends on the rest of the intake. Fiber, like almost everything else, can be abused.
• Adjust mealtimes and size to your schedule. Don't exercise or sleep on a stomach loaded with heavy food.
• Cut down on animal protein, particularly red meat with its high level of saturated fats.
• Try to put meals together with a view to balance—different food groups and complementary attributes, such as something high in iron with a companion (or sauce) rich in vitamin C.
• Be alert to the need to keep sodium/potassium and calcium/phosphorous levels in proportion. Check labels for sodium (salt) and phosphates. Cool water is far and away the best refresher.
• Vitamin and mineral supplements in normal dosages do no harm, but a well-balanced diet with an emphasis on fresh fruit, vegetables, and grains for most healthy people (who are not extremely active or under great stress) is usually sufficient by itself. Try to evaluate the weaknesses (whether from habit or geography) in your diet when selecting the right supplements.
• If it works and you feel well, stick with it. Don't experiment with a new regime for the sake of trying a fad. A change in lifestyle may well require a change in diet.

These ideas may sound obvious, but how many of us really follow them? For top athletes, especially as they mature, proper nutrition is no longer a luxury. I hope their example and advice will help you to live longer and more healthfully.

# Index

# ABOUT THE AUTHOR

Jane Wilkens Michael is a contributing editor of *Town & Country* magazine. Her articles have also appeared in *The New York Times, International Herald Tribune, Harper's Bazaar,* and *Cosmopolitan.* She lives in New York City with her husband and two sons.